KT-368-027

WATER EXERCISES

WORKOUTS WITH THE AQUA NOODLE

Tomihiro Shimizu/Noriko Tachikawa

Michael DeToia (ed.)

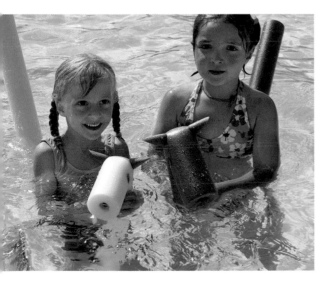
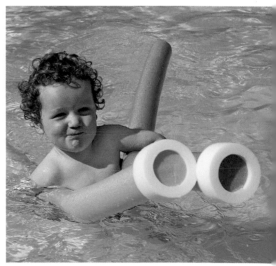

Meyer & Meyer Sport

British Library Cataloguing in Publication Data
A catalogue record for this book is available from the British Library

Water Exercises
Workouts with the Aqua Noodle
Tomihiro Shimizu / Noriko Tachikawa
Michael DeToia (ed.)
Maidenhead: Meyer & Meyer Sport (UK) Ltd., 2004
2nd Edition 2009
ISBN 978-1-84126-143-0

All rights reserved, especially the right to copy and distribute, including the translation rights. No part of this work may be reproduced – including by photocopy, microfilm or any other means – processed, stored electronically, copied or distributed in any form whatsoever without the written permission of the publisher.

© 2004 by Meyer & Meyer Sport (UK) Ltd.
2nd Edition 2009

Aachen, Adelaide, Auckland, Budapest, Cape Town, Graz, Indianapolis,
Maidenhead, New York, Olten (CH), Singapore, Toronto
Member of the World
Sport Publishers' Association (WSPA)
www.w-s-p-a.org

Printed and bound by: B.O.S.S Druck und Medien GmbH, Germany
ISBN 978-1-84126-143-0
E-Mail: verlag@m-m-sports.com
www.m-m-sports.com

TABLE OF CONTENTS

Chapter I: Theory

Chapter II : The Aqua Noodle Workout Program

FOREWORD
BY THE AUTHORS

I am very happy, thanks to the cooperation of our various colleagues worldwide, improved medical techniques and natural healing methods - especially underwater movement therapy and Balneotherapy - that our book will appear in bookshops in the German- and English-speaking world.

Japan´s economic situation is currently stagnant. This situation has given us time to think. The Japanese have a greater appreciation of life´s spiritual values rather than its material ones. This, in turn, has influenced the development of natural healing methods, therefore, creating a higher interest for relaxation techniques. Water as a form of therapy integrates both "workout" and gentle relaxation. I hope that the development of aquatic therapy and exercise will be appreciated also in English-speaking countries.

I would like to thank Michael DeToia from DEHAG ACADEMY for the realization of the book, Mrs. Heintz for the book corrections, and Daniela DeToia for the translation into the English language.

Niigata, Japan, December 2003   Tomihiro Shimizu
                                       Noriko Tachikawa

FOREWORD
BY THE EDITOR

It is stunning that despite the popularity of the aqua noodle there is no detailed collection of exercises for this classic modern Aquaworkout equipment. All the more we are looking forward to presenting the great line-up of ideas all around the aqua noodle and the animating illustrations of the Japanese authors Tomihiro Shimizu and Noriko Tachikawa. This book should be an outstanding source for instructors and all users of the aqua noodle for a safe and efficient Aquaworkout. Fun is guaranteed in the playfully challenging, wet medium: Water!

Michael DeToia
Chairman, DEHAG ACADEMY

The Aqua Noodle: THE All-round-equipment for Workouts in Water

The colorful aqua noodle is the least expensive and most multi-functional all-round equipment for the water workout. The funny aqua noodle has displaced the classical float and it provides unlimited opportunities through its flexibility, which reaches to the point that one can make a knot in it. By cutting through the middle of the noodle you can make two shorter so called aqua-noodle sticks from it, that can be used by themselves or in pairs.

When you workout with a fixated handle you should keep in mind not to stay in one grip-position too long. This could lead to pain in the area of your hands and forearm/elbow, because of an overload that can lead to a tennis or golfers-elbow. The cause of this rising problem is the fact that the handle on the noodle is not ergonomic. The diameter of the noodle is simply too large. This is why it is also senseless to cut the sticks into half again in order to use these parts as dumbbells.

First of all the aqua noodle can be used as an ideal backup. One can compare it to the situation on a sling table. The faster you move the noodle through the water, the more you work with the water resistance and the more power is applied. The slower the movement becomes, the more the improvement of stabilization and posture is in the foreground. Working your arms and legs, working in a sitting position, diagonally or along the noodle, working on your stabilization with one or two noodles or even standing on it and using the stretching effects above the surface, everything is possible with the aqua noodle.

Interesting to know: Initially this equipment was designed for chair-gymnastics on land with senior citizens…

Michael DeToia, editor
November 2008

CHAPTER 1: THEORY

1 AQUA WELLNESS

Since the beginning of the ´60s the word "wellness" in the USA and Europe has been a new expression of the health conscious person. Being healthy is not only just "not being sick" but the positive feeling of body wellness. Everybody should actively care enough about his body and mind so he can be healthy and stay healthy.

Aqua Wellness is a word composed of "aqua", "well-being" and "fitness" and also the leading physical movement through water: water for wellness. In other words, using water to stay healthy and fit and enjoy a good feeling.

Figure 1 shows aqua wellness in three different aspects – the influence of the intensity of the exercise and physical activity: aquatic therapy, aquatic exercise and aquatic sport. Aquatic rehabilitation belongs to the aquatic therapy category.

Where in the training process can the aqua noodle be applied in aqua wellness? The aqua noodle can be introduced in all kinds of aquatic therapy, aquatic exercise and aquatic sport territories: in the swimming pool, the lake, the ocean, the river or in sports, in leisure programs, in activities for therapy and for fitness improvement.

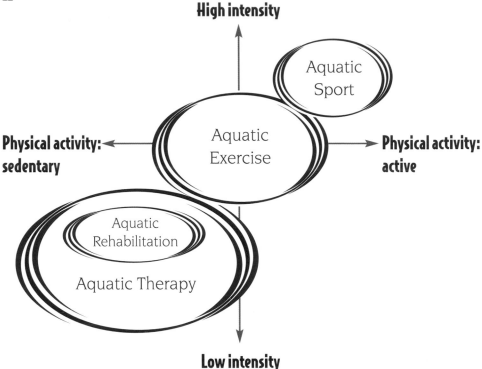

Fig. 1 Three main aspects of aqua wellness, influenced by intensity level and physical activity (Tomihiro Shimizu)

The swimming pool has been chosen by students and adults mainly to learn the swimming technique and to improve the swimming art. Today we see more and more old and young people going to the swimming pool for water gymnastic exercises. That means that in the future the swimming pool will be used more for aquatic exercises and aquatic therapy not only for a swim. Therefore, the aqua noodle will be used even more frequently in the future.

As indispensable as the polystyrene board is to learning to swim, so will the aqua noodle be nessecary for aqua gymnastics in the future.

2 THE AQUA NOODLE PROPERTIES AND ACCESSORIES

2.1 The Name of the Aqua Noodle

I have realized that in the USA, Germany, Switzerland, France and Spain the aqua noodle is used in leisure activities, therapy programs and in training for groups of various ages. The name of the tool was always different: Aqua noodle, Pool-noodle, aqualog, aquaball, fun-noodle, aquatube and so on. In this book, we will use the term aqua noodle. I hope the word aqua noodle will be used in the aqua gymnastic language for years to come throughout the world, like pasta or asian noodles.

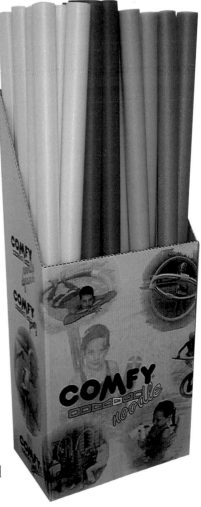

2.2 The Properties of the Aqua Noodle

The aqua noodle as shown in Illustration 1 is a swim cylinder. The properties are put together in Table 1. The quality is different according to the manufacturor, but the length is about 160cm and 7cm in diameter. The lift power is about 5 to 6kg. The exercise program, depending on the purpose, can be put together in a creative form. The aqua noodle can be bought in several colours and provides a nice atmosphere.

The material is soft, elastic, smooth to hold on and to bend. The aqua noodle can motivate the user to playfully exercise with it.

Tab. 1: Properties of the aqua noodle

Shape	Cylinder
Material	Polyethylene foam (PE) free of FCKW- & HFCKW
Size	160cm x 7cm (ø)
Weight	c. 150 g
Buoyancy	c. 6 kg

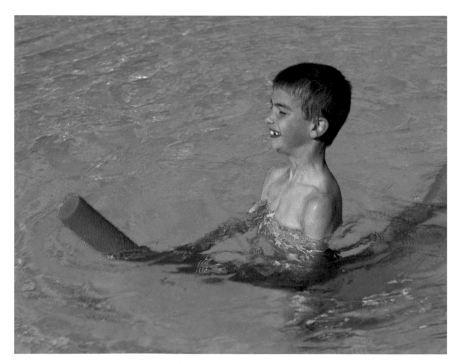

Illustration 1: Shape of the aqua noodle

2.3   Noodle Sticks : The Half Noodle

The aqua noodle can be cut in the middle with a carpet cutter. The half aqua noodle is known as a noodle stick. The half noodle is 80cm length and the lifting power is about 3kg. The procedure is very simple. Just mark it in the middle, and you can easily cut through with a knife. This special knife can be bought in a hardware store. Make sure when you cut the aqua noodle, the cut is vertical and done in one cut. (Illustration 2/3). The half aqua noodles are not only for children but also for beginners and for many exercises that will be mentioned later.

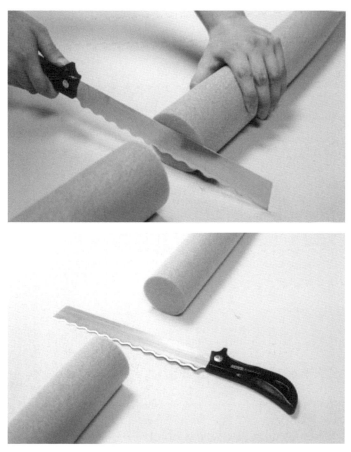

Illustration 2/3: Cutting the aqua noodle

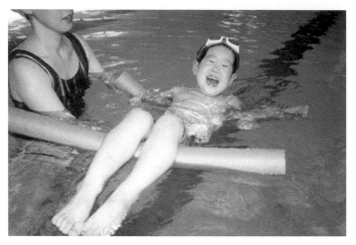

Illustration 4: Using the aqua noodle

2.4 Accessories: Connectors

The aqua noodle can be connected with connectors (Illustration 5) made of polyethylene (PE), the material that is also used in making the aqua noodle.

With pieces connected to the aqua noodle, there are options to make a raft (Illustration 6), a hoop to jump through (Illustration 8).

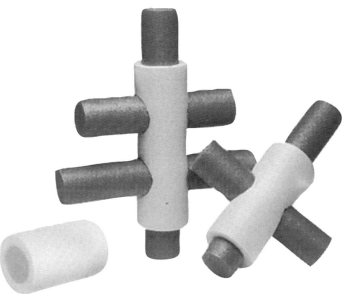

Illustration 5: Connectors

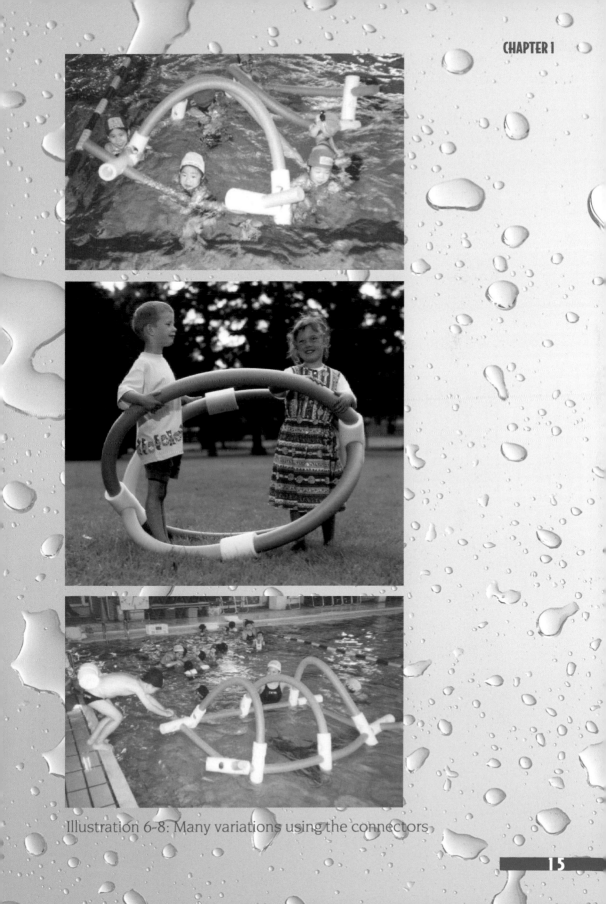

Illustration 6-8: Many variations using the connectors

2.5. Storage

To keep the aqua noodle in good condition, it is best to put it in a ball carriage (Illustration 9) or a basket (Illustration 10).

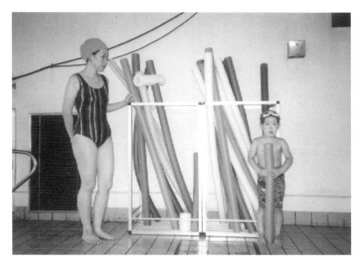

Illustration 9: Ball carriage

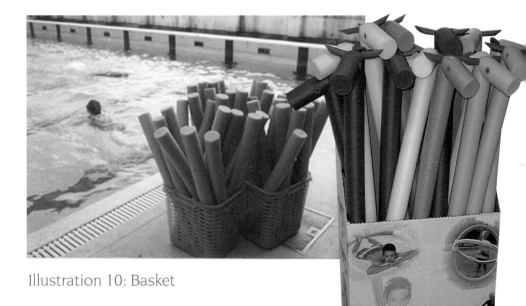

Illustration 10: Basket

3   APPLICATIONS FOR THE AQUA NOODLE

3.1   The Basic Characteristics of the Aqua Noodle

The three basic characteristics of the aqua noodle exercises are: facilitating, assisting and resisting movements.

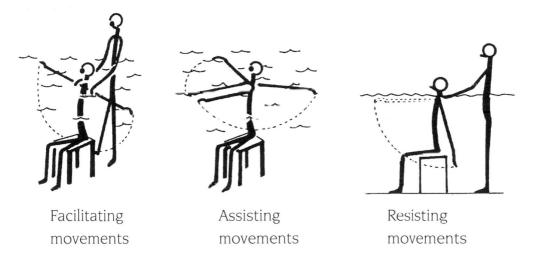

Facilitating movements

Assisting movements

Resisting movements

Fig. 2: The 3 basic characteristics

Facilitating Movements

The aqua noodle is supported by the buoyancy of the water. That is why the exercises will be performed almost without gravity. Most of the exercises belong in this category. Many of the exercises with the aqua noodle are executed as a basic form.

Assisting Movements

The angle of the buoyancy direction and the movement direction is mostly 90°, while the movement is parallel to the surface of the water. As the postural muscle system is supported by buoyancy, water creates a better situation for any kind of movement.

Resisting movements

The movement direction is opposite to the direction of the force of buoyancy. This makes the extensor muscular system stronger (see Illustration 13).

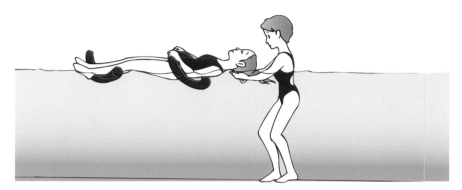

Illustration 11: Facilitating movements with the aqua noodle

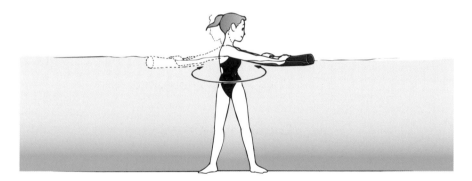

Illustration 12: Movement support with the aqua noodle

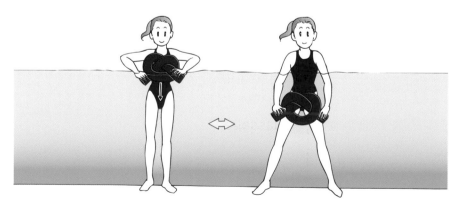

Illustration 13: Resisting movements with the aqua noodle

3.2   Single, Partner or Group Exercises

Exercises with the aqua noodle can be practiced alone, with a partner or in a group: 1, 2 or even 3 aqua noodles can be used. The aqua noodle can be changed from a cylinder to a ring with a connector bringing both ends together. Both forms also can be combined.

3.3   Training Goals and Objectives

The goals for training with the aqua noodle can be split into seven areas (see Fig. 3). In the practical part of this book each exercise will be explained in detail.

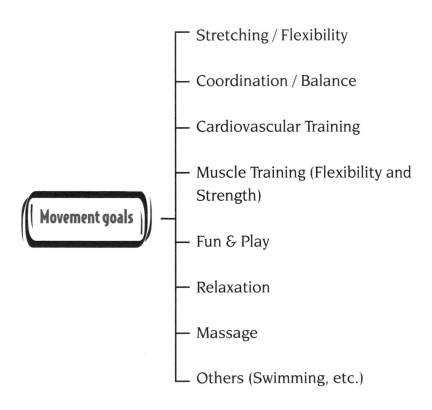

Fig. 3: Movement goals using the aqua noodle (T. Shimizu, 1998)

Stretching

Most stretching exercises follow the first basic characteristic of facilitating movements. The person will be carried by the aqua noodle and led through a stretching program, for example see Illustration 14 and 15 for an exercise for stretching the gluteal muscles. Illustration 16 and 17 are for the waistline and Illustration 18 and 19 target the hips. These exercises are also recomended for back problems.

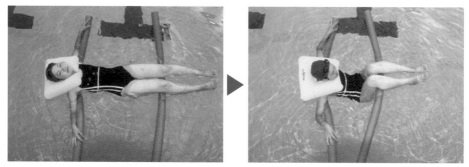

Illustration 14/15: Stretching the lower back

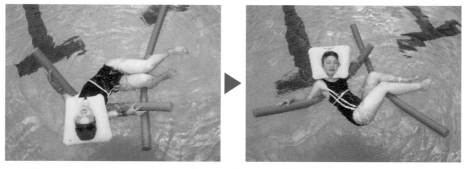

Illustration 16/17: Stretching the waistline

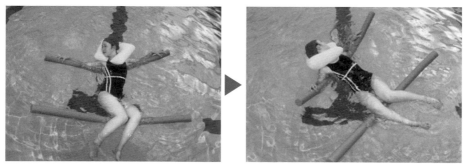

Illustration 18/19: Stretching the hips

Coordination (Balance)

The aqua noodle can be of assistance in keeping your balance. It can also be a big help for most unstable positions.

Moving in water, the center of gravity and the center of buoyancy are constantly changing due to buoyancy, waves, turbulence and resistance. In this complex situation, balance must be constantly corrected. This is a good exercise for coordination, training the vestibular system in the ear, the good feeling for movements, the brain, and the visual and hearing systems. Illustration 20 and 21 show a coordination exercise. With outstretched arms, the person puts the aqua noodle behind his back and pulls out from the center position to the side.

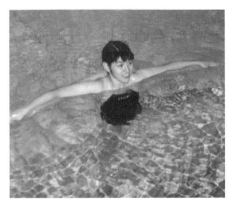 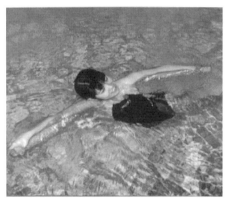

Illustration 20/21: Coordination exercise

Cardiovascular Training

Training your heart and blood vessels with long movements with a low load will improve cardiovascular functions.

Illustration 22 shows an example of this kind of exercise. This training should take 20 to 40 minutes and is compensating

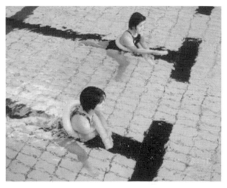

Illustration 22: Endurance

for any imbalances and differences between the right and left parts of your body.

Muscle Training (Flexibility and Strength)

During strength exrercises, the aqua noodle is pressed down against buoyancy. Illustration 23 and 24 show this exercise; the person takes the aqua noodle behind the back, then stretches and bends the arms. This is an exercise to strengthen the arm extensors and the muscles of the lower arm and the rear parts of the shoulder girdle (especially m. trapezius).

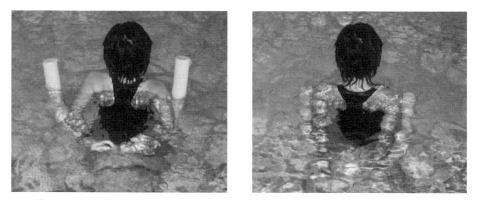

Illustration 23/24: Strengthening the arms

Fun & Play

The exercises with the aqua noodle are mainly for communication, variation and to reduce stress. The exercises are similar to endurance and strength exercises, but the main point here is the fun factor. Illustration 25 shows an exercise: the locomotive.

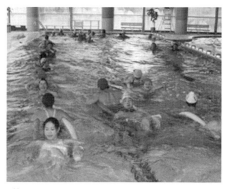

Illustration 25: Fun & Play

Relaxation and Massage

The exercises are mainly practiced on the water surface. The aqua noodles are very helpful for these exercises.

Illustration 26 shows an exercise program that helps you to relax with an aqua noodle and a swim collar with music. Illustration 27 shows an exercise for relaxing in a group.

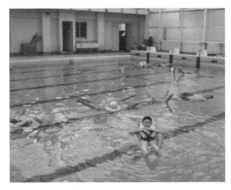
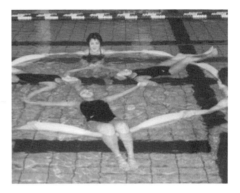

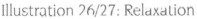
Illustration 26/27: Relaxation

Other Areas for Application of the Aqua Noodle

The aqua noodle can also be used in the aquagymnastics aspect, for example, for getting used to the water or learning how to swim. Illustration 28 shows one swimming exercise (crawl: leg movement), Illustration 29 shows another exercise for crawl swimming. There are many other possibilities.

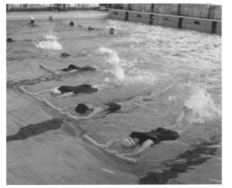
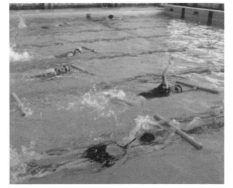

Illustration 28: Crawl: leg movement
Illustration 29: Crawl: special drills with the aqua noodle

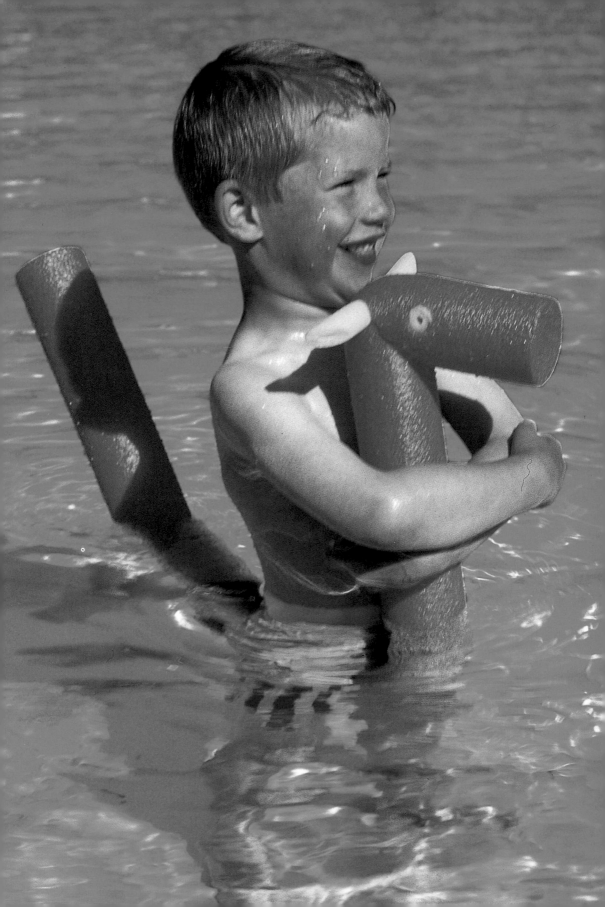

CHAPTER II:
THE AQUA NOODLE WORKOUT PROGRAM

- Stretching
- Coordination (Balance)
- Cardio Training
- Toning: Muscle Training for Strength and Flexibility
- Fun & Play
- Massage and Relaxation

Explanation of the Exercise

Name and number of the exercise

Goal of the movement

Picture of the exercise

Explanation of the exercise

Variations

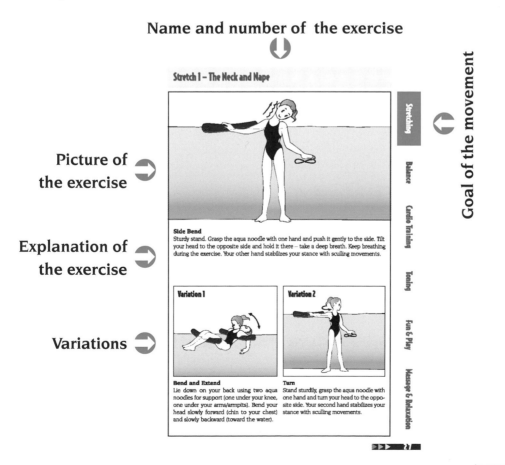

Stretch I – The Neck and Nape

Stretching
Balance
Cardio Training
Toning
Fun & Play
Massage & Relaxation

Side Bend
Sturdy stand. Grasp the aqua noodle with one hand and push it gently to the side. Tilt your head to the opposite side and hold it there – take a deep breath. Keep breathing during the exercise. Your other hand stabilizes your stance with sculling movements.

Variation 1

Variation 2

Bend and Extend
Lie down on your back using two aqua noodles for support (one under your knee, one under your arms/armpits). Bend your head slowly forward (chin to your chest) and slowly backward (toward the water).

Turn
Stand sturdily, grasp the aqua noodle with one hand and turn your head to the opposite side. Your second hand stabilizes your stance with sculling movements.

Coordination

Agility Training

Toning

Fun & Play

Massage & Relaxation

STRETCHING

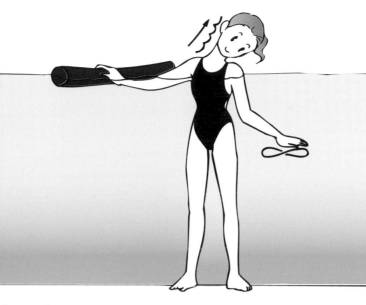

Side Bend

Sturdy stance. Grasp the aqua noodle with one hand and push it gently to the side. Tilt your head to the opposite side and hold it there – take a deep breath. Keep breathing during the exercise. Your other hand stabilizes your stance with sculling movements.

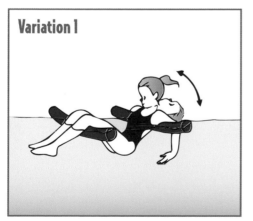

Variation 1

Bend and Extend

Lie down on your back using two aqua noodles for support (one under your knee, one under your arms/armpits). Bend your head slowly forward (chin to your chest) and slowly backward (toward the water).

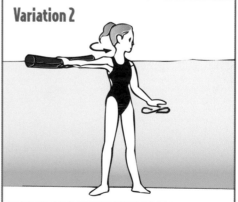

Variation 2

Turn

Stand sturdily, grasp the aqua noodle with one hand and turn your head to the opposite side. Your second hand stabilizes your stance with sculling movements.

Stretch 2 - The Shoulder

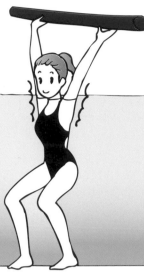

Mobilisation of the shoulder

Stand sturdily. The shoulders are in the water, grasp the aqua noodle and bring your arms straight up in the air. Leave your shoulder girdle in the water.

To intensify the exercise, stretch your arms slowly behind your ears. To increase the stretch further bring your arms together.

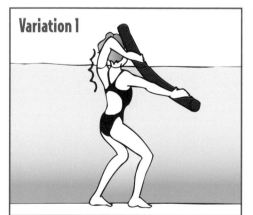

Variation 1

Variation 2

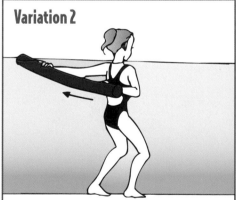

**Movement of the elbow
(shoulder and the side)**
Grasp the aqua noodle with your hands, arms straight up in the air, bend one arm behind your head and bring your other arm straight down (alternating sides).

**Elbow stretch back
(shoulder and chest)**
Grasp the aqua noodle behind your back, bend one arm and stretch the other, alternating sides. Leave shoulder girdle under the water.

Stretch 3 – The Chest

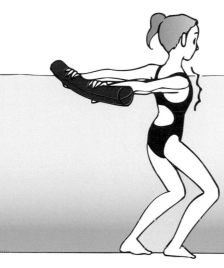

Chest and shoulder

Lay your hands behind your back on the aqua noodle and tilt your upper body to the front. The closer your hands are the more intense the stretch becomes. To increase the exercise push the aqua noodle together with your hands.

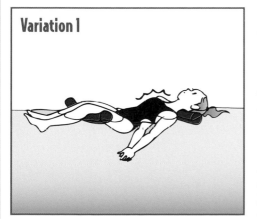

Variation 1

Chest and shoulder

Lie down on your back using two aqua noodles for support, fold your hands behind your back and stretch your arms down. Be careful to keep your balance.

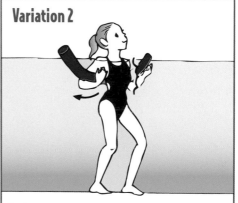

Variation 2

Chest

Bring the aqua noodle behind your back and put it under your arms. Slowly straighten your upper body and tilt it slightly backward. Do not overextend.

Coordination Cardio Training Toning Fun & Play Massage & Relaxation

Stretch 4 – The Back

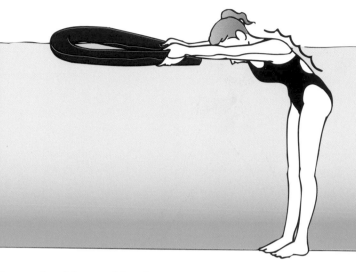

Arms, shoulder and back

Take a sturdy stance. Hold both ends of the aqua noodle and bring them together.
Round your back: Head and upper body are tilted forward, take a deep breath.

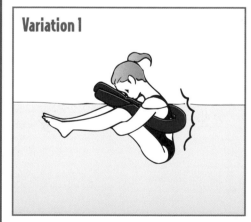

Variation 1

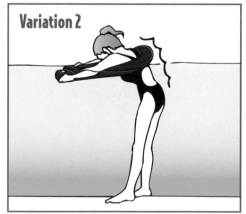

Variation 2

Chest and lower back

Squeeze the aqua noodle under your arms, bring your legs up and embrace them. In case this is too hard, the hands can be laid upon the knees. Keep an eye on your balance.

Upper back

Squeeze the aqua noodle under your arms behind your back and take hold of both ends. Tilt your head and upper body forward.

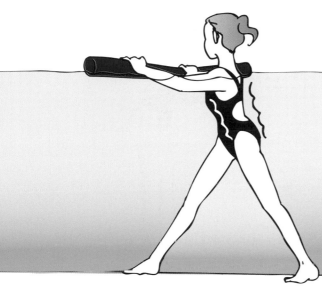

Obliques

Lay your hands on the aqua noodle and turn your upper body to the side (using a bigger range of motion take your hips with you and pick up your heel – sturdy torso). Alternate sides.

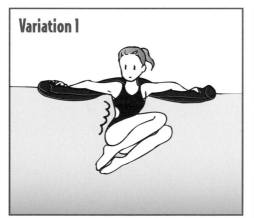

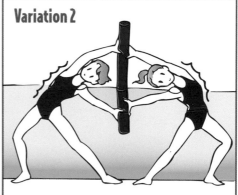

Variation 1

Variation 2

Obliques

Lay your arms on the aqua noodle, crouch your legs and tilt your legs side to side like the twist.

Flank

Two people stand next to each other in a squat. The aqua noodle is vertical in the water. Both people tilt their upper bodies toward the aqua noodle and grasp it with both hands.

Stretch 6 – The Hip

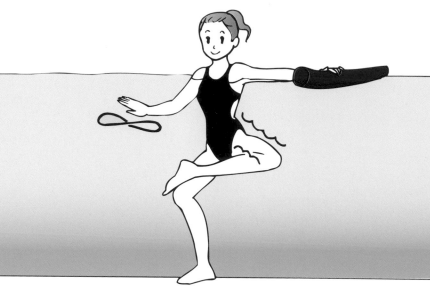

Hip and gluteus

Take hold of the aqua noodle with one hand, lay one foot on top of the other leg and keep the knee out. Balance with the other hand.

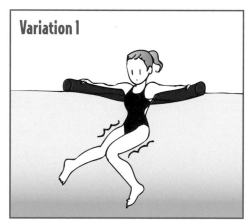

Variation 1

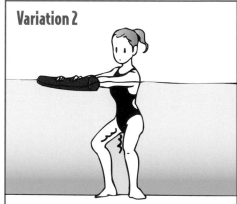

Variation 2

Abductors

Bring the aqua noodle behind your back and lay your arms on top. Squeeze your knees together and turn your lower legs out. Now hold.

Adductors

Lay your hands on top of the aqua noodle, which is in front of you, straddle it. Bend your knees slightly. Slowly move your knees out.

Stretch 7 – The Thigh

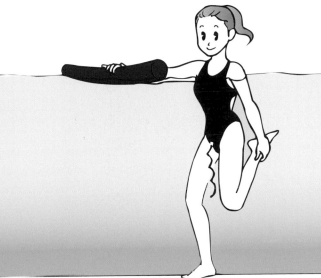

Stretching the thigh
Lay one hand on the aqua noodle for balance, the other hand pulls the opposite foot toward your buttocks.

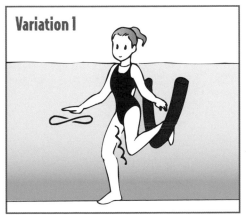

Variation 1

Stretching the thigh
Lay one foot on the aqua noodle behind your back and hold it there. The aqua noodle should not be too high because of the buoyancy of the water. Do not over-extend.

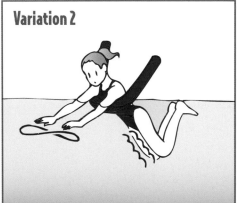

Variation 2

Stretching the thigh
Lie with your stomach on the aqua noodle, bend your knees and pull your feet toward your buttocks.
Your hands stabilize the exercise. Your hip must be extended. This is an advanced exercise.

Stretching
Coordination
Cardio Training
Toning
Fun & Play
Massage & Relaxation

Stretch 8 – The Gluteus and Hamstrings

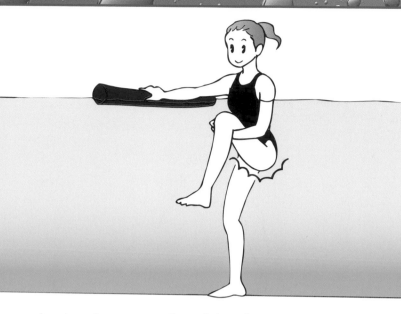

Lay one hand on the aqua noodle and the other under your knee. Now pull your knee toward your stomach and hold (exhale).

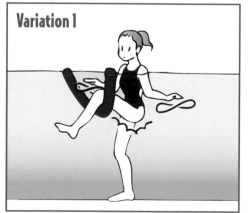

Variation 1

Lay the aqua noodle under your knee, pull your knee towards your stomach for an intense stretch. This is an advanced exercise due to the high buoyancy of the water.

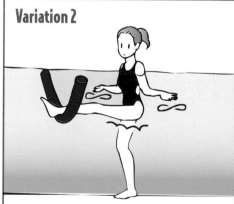

Variation 2

Lay an extended leg in front of you on the aqua noodle. This stretches your gluteus and hamstrings. If you are small or have back problems, this exercise should be done with caution due to the high buoyancy of the water.

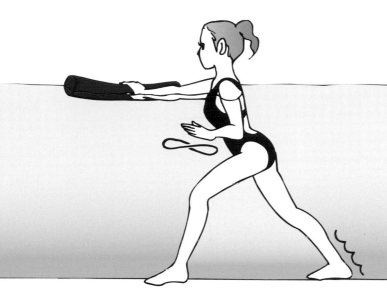

The calf and the hip flexors

Lay one hand on the aqua noodle to stabilize your stance. Lunge to the front, your front leg is bent and your hip is flexed. Your back foot stays on the floor. Your other hand stabilizes your stand with sculling movements.

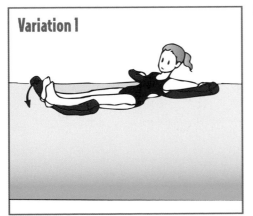

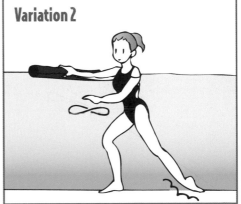

Variation 1

Variation 2

Calf and shin

Lie down backward on two aqua noodles, pull your feet toward your nose or stretch them, hold them or make circles.

Shin and hip-flexor

Lunge to the front, lay one hand on the aqua noodle and extend your hip and your foot in the back and hold it there.

COORDINATION

Coordination 1 – Surfing

Stretching

Coordination

Cardio Training

Toning

Fun & Play

Massage & Relaxation

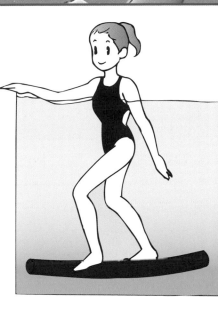

Balance with both feet on the aqua noodle. Move, walk and turn on the aqua noodle as if you were surfing. You can hold onto the edge of the pool for support.

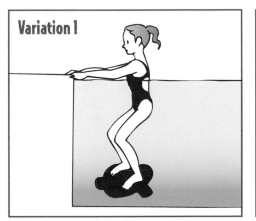

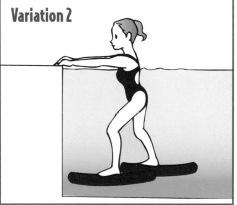

The circus
Stand on the knotted aqua noodle. It is easier to balance on the aqua noodle with slightly flexed hips and bent knees.

Skiing
Stand on two aqua noodles and move to the front. Using a long aqua noodle this exercise becomes advanced.

Coordination 2 – Balance the Object

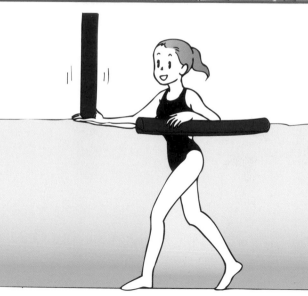

Put an object on your head or on your hand and try to balance it. If you can manage this in the water, it is even easier for you on land. The picture on top shows the following: Put an aqua noodle on your hand and try to walk. For an advanced workout: Balance an aqua noodle on your finger tips and try to walk.

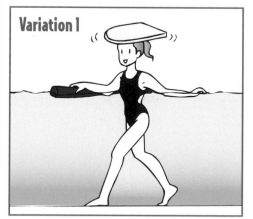

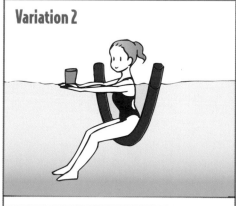

Perfect posture

Lay one hand on the aqua noodle, put a board on your head and try to move forward. You can use other objects or vary your starting position. Walk forward and keep an eye on your balance.

The perfect sitting position

Sit on the aqua noodle, hold an object in your hand and try to keep your balance. This exercise is a challenge. (The picture shows a person holding a cup filled with water in the palms of his hands.)

Coordination 3 – Perfect Posture: the Vertical

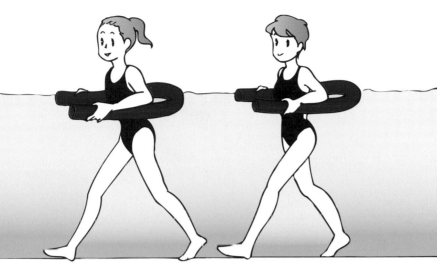

Put the aqua noodle under your arms, take hold of the ends, walk forward and keep your balance.

Variation 1

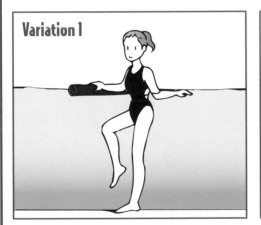

Flamingo

Grasp the aqua noodle with one hand, stand on one leg and hold it there. Move the other leg and keep your balance.

Variation 2

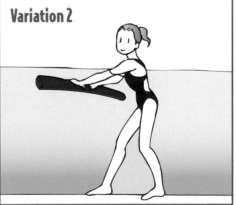

Standing

Stay in one spot and move the aqua noodle around, changing the position of your upper body without moving your feet. Keep your balance each time you change your position.

Stretching

Coordination

Cardio Training

Toning

Fun & Play

Massage & Relaxation

Coordination 4 – Perfect Posture: Sitting

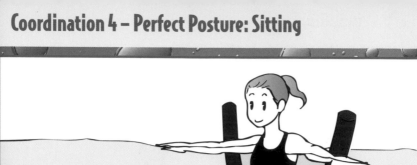

Sit on the aqua noodle without touching the floor (in suspension). Your hands support you to keep your balance.

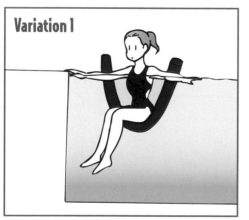

Variation 1

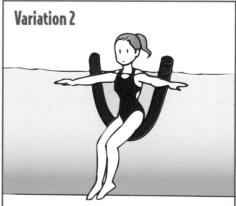

Variation 2

Hold onto the edge of the pool to modify the exercise. This is easier than keeping your balance with the help of your hands (sculling movements).

Beginners should touch the floor with their toes, which stabilizes the stance.

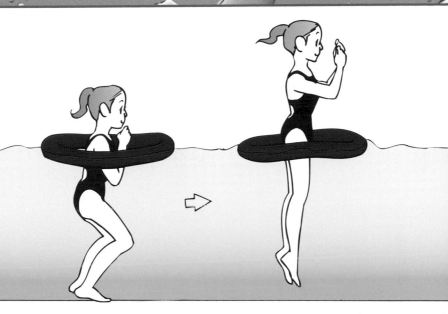

Connect two aqua noodles to a ring (with a connector) and jump in the ring, up and down, moving forward. Keep your balance. In case you lose your balance, hold onto the aqua noodle.

Variation 1

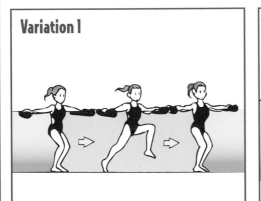

Jumping to the side
Hold onto two aqua noodles with each hand, push off from the floor and jump to the side. Try to land carefully on the floor (joint-free movement).

Variation 2

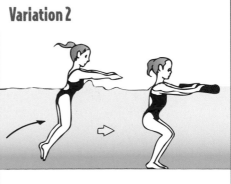

The bunny jump
Squat down and jump towards the aqua noodle in front of you. Land carefully with both feet on the floor (joint-free movement).

Stretching

Coordination

Cardio Training

Toning

Fun & Play

Massage & Relaxation

Coordination 6 – Suspension

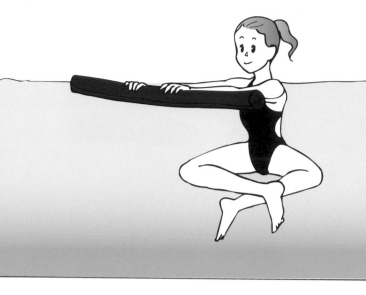

There are several different starting positions possible in the water. The picture shows a person holding onto the aqua noodle with both hands. Sit cross-legged, keeping the body vertical.

Variation:
Hold the aqua noodle with only one hand. Keep your balance with your other hand. Extend your legs in deep water.

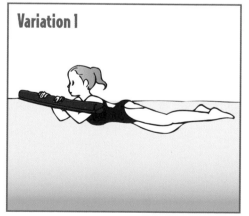

Variation 1

Prone
Hold onto the aqua noodle with both hands in a prone position and try to keep your body in a horizontal position by using your legs.

Variation 2

Supine
Put an aqua noodle under each arm in a supine position keeping your body in a horizontal line.

Coordination 7 – Suspension 2

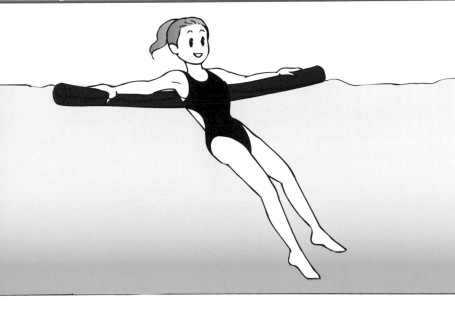

Lie in a supine position on the aqua noodle and twist your body so that you are in a diagonal position.

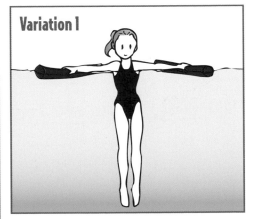

Variation 1

Cross
Your body is in a vertical line. This is not easy in the water. Try not to hold onto the aqua noodle too tightly.

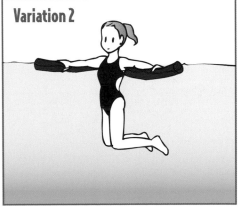

Variation 2

Bent knees
Bend your knees, keeping your torso straight so that your feet are in the direction of your spine. This is an advanced exercise because the starting position is not very stable.

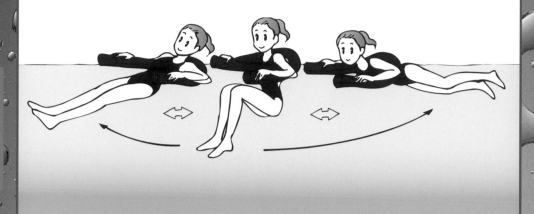

Rocking your pelvis

Lie in a supine position on the aqua noodle. Now, move your pelvis over the vertical position back in a prone position. This changes your center of gravity. This is an advanced exercise (not suitable for people with back problems).

Variation 1

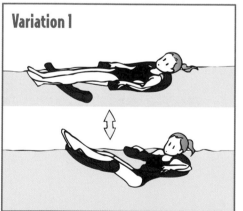

Variation 2

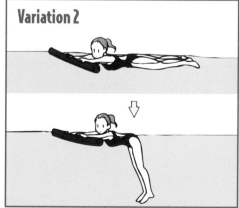

V-position

Lie in a supine position on the aqua noodle and put a second aqua noodle under your knees so your body is in a horizontal position. Now tilt your pelvis down so you are in a v-position and extend your pelvis back to the starting position. Do not jerk your body!

Lay both hands on the aqua noodle in a prone position. Now, bend your pelvis so your legs are in a vertical position and your feet touch the floor. Your stomach muscles should be working hard during this exercise. The exercise is easier when the feet do not touch the floor. You also have the possibility of keeping your feet together.

Coordination 9 – The Turn

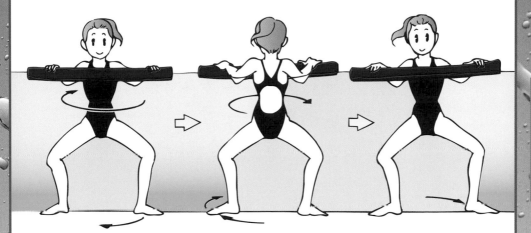

Lay both hands on the aqua noodle and turn your whole body around. Turn left or turn right (alternate), but do not turn too fast.

Variation 1

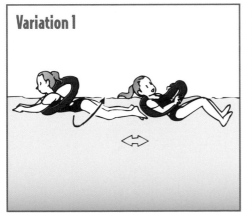

Turning horizontal

Put the aqua noodle formed like a ring around your body. Now, turn your body from the prone position to the supine position. Use your hands for balance.

Variation 2

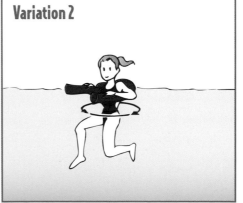

Vertical position

Put the aqua noodle under your arms and turn your whole body around. Your upper body should stay vertical during this exercise. Use your hands and legs for balance.

Coordination 10 – The Combination

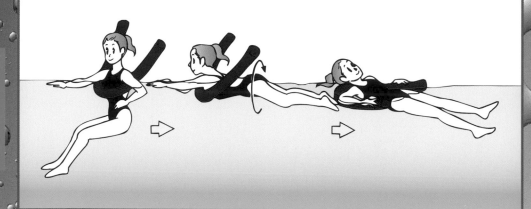

Put the aqua noodle under your arms so the ends are behind you. This is a combination of the vertical stance over to the supine position with the help of a turn. The picture shows the person in a vertical position, moving the pelvis up so the person is in a prone position. Now turning the whole body around to the supine position. This exercise is not always suitable for therapy or beginners.

Variation 1

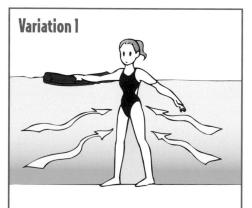

Against the water
Lay one hand on the aqua noodle and try to keep a stabilized stance against the current. The other participants produce the waves.

Variation 2

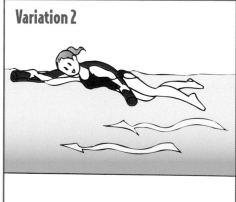

In the current of the water
Go with the current and try to keep stable.

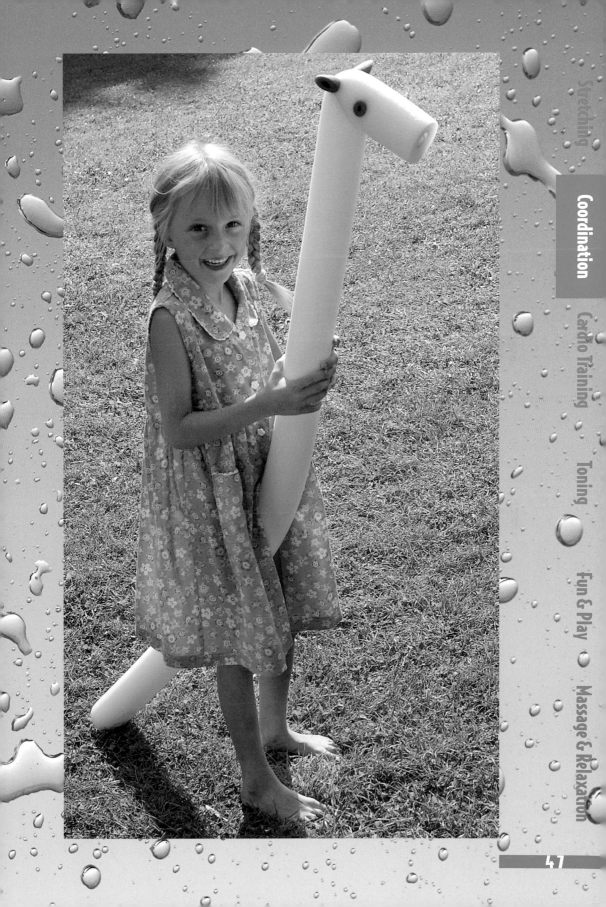

Stretching

Coordination

Cardio Training

Toning

Fun & Play

Massage & Relaxation

Stretching

Coordination

Cardio Training

Combined

Fun & Play

Massage & Relaxation

CARDIO TRAINING

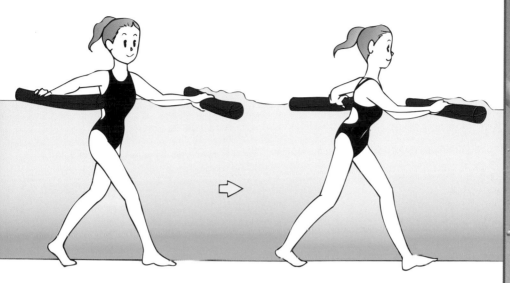

Walk forward with one aqua noodle in each hand for support, either next to your body or in front of you for more resistance. You can begin the exercise from different starting positions. If the water is too shallow, tilt your upper body forward, be aware of your posture.

Variation 1

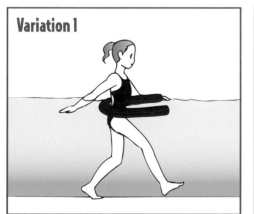

Walking backward
Beginners should lean backward against the aqua noodle.

Variation 2

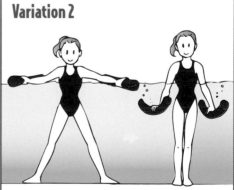

Walking sideways
Place each hand on an aqua noodle and move the aqua noodle up and down, which makes the exercise harder.

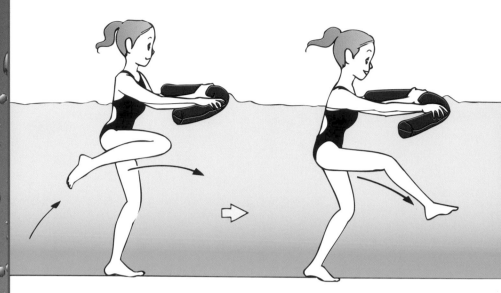

Hurdle-race with big steps

Hold onto the aqua noodle, which is in front of you, pull your knee up and jump over an imagined hurdle.

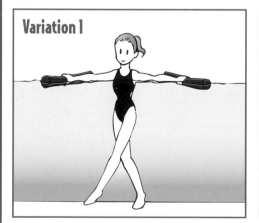

Variation 1

Step cross

Place each hand on an aqua noodle for support and walk forward with crossed legs. Watch out for abduction and adduction.

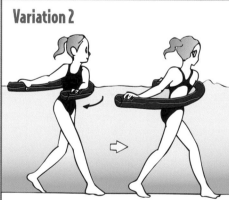

Variation 2

Turn step

Walk forward by only turning your upper body side to side, which means make a step with your left leg and turn your body to the left side at the same time.

Cardio Training 3 – Jogging

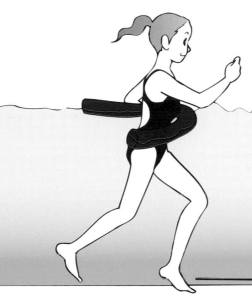

Jog in the water by touching the floor with your feet. You can use the aqua noodle for support or for resistance in front of your stomach. It is possible to run forward, backward, to the side, make turns or do some figures.

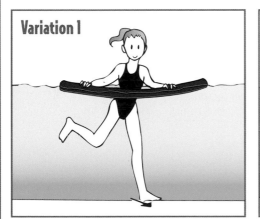

Variation 1

Parting your legs
Jog to the side, keeping your legs apart. During the exercise, hold onto the aqua noodle and bend your knee or pull your foot toward your buttocks.

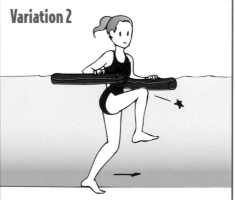

Variation 2

Jumping with the knee up
Hold onto one aqua noodle on each side, pulling your knees up to the aqua noodle and run forward.

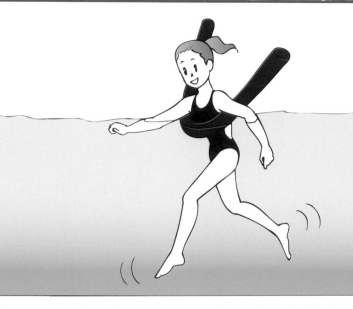

Put the aqua noodle under your arms so the ends are behind you. Now, jog forward without touching the floor. Find your own best starting position. Use your arms for support by scooping the water.

Variation 1

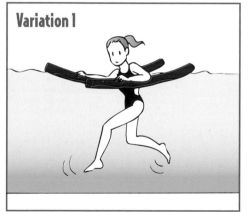

Lean on the aqua noodles (one on each side) and jog forward without touching the floor. In doing so, the buoyancy and the resistance are high because you are using two aqua noodles.

Variation 2

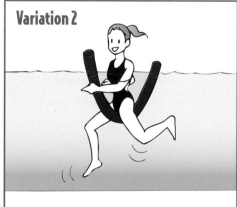

Sit on the aqua noodle. Do not hold on tight to the aqua noodle and try to jog forward. Keep your back straight.

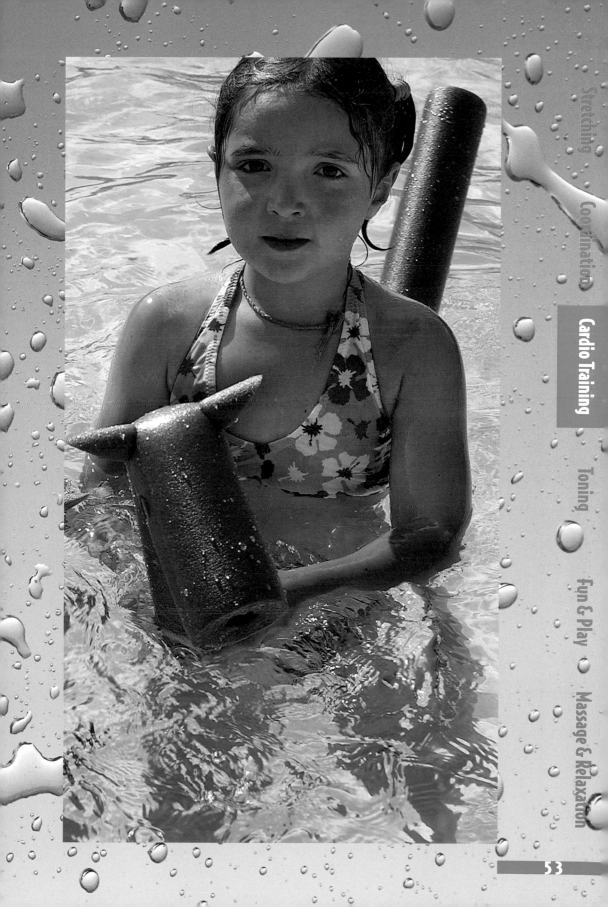

TONING:
MUSCLE TRAINING (STRENGTH AND FLEXIBILITY)

Stretching

Coordination

Cardio Training

Toning

Fun & Play

Massage & Relaxation

Toning 1 – Half-turn

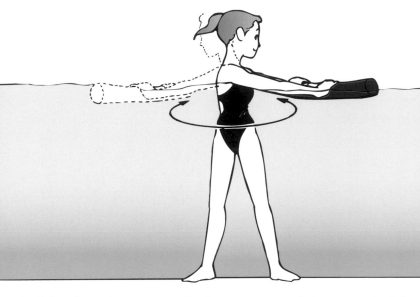

Lay both hands on the aqua noodle. Turn your torso all the way to the left or right side. When using a small range of motion, keep your stance stable and turn your body keeping your torso upright. When using a larger range of motion turn your pelvis in the same direction and pick up your heel in the back keeping your torso stable. Tip for older participants: Do not turn too fast because lower back problems or dizziness might occur.

Variation 1

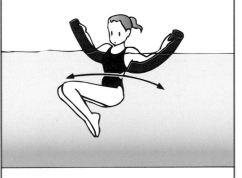

Buttocks

Squeeze the aqua noodle from the back under your arms. Bend both knees and tilt them to the right and to the left. This exercise must be performed with caution to protect the lower back.

Variation 2

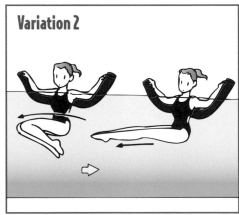

Abdominal

Squeeze the aqua noodle from the back under your arms, bend your knees, tilt them to the side and extend your legs slowly. No jerky movements or it will strain the lower back.

Toning 2 – Twist with Knee

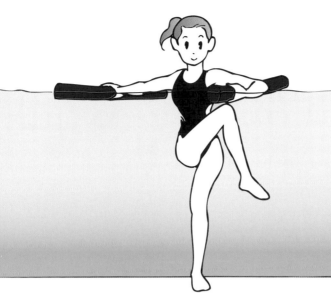

Place each hand on one aqua noodle. Diagonal movement: Lift your right knee diagonal to your left hand and, at the same time, move your left hand to your right arm. Perform this exercise slowly.

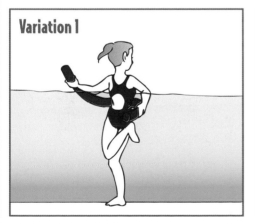

Variation 1

Twist with your heel to your buttocks
Put your hands on the aqua noodle which is in front of you, bend your left knee toward your buttocks and move the right end of the aqua noodle toward your left foot behind you. Do not turn your head too far.

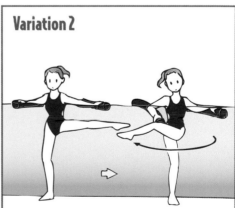

Variation 2

Twist with straight legs
Hold one aqua noodle on each side, extend your left leg to the side, then cross it to the right side and move the right end of the aqua noodle toward your leg.

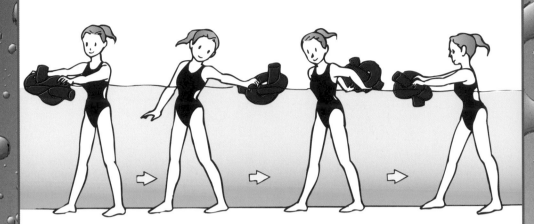

Turn on your own axis. This exercise is different than the half-turn around your own axis. The picture shows the body rotation. Move the knotted aqua noodle around your body as far away as possible. Do not overextend your back.

Variation 1

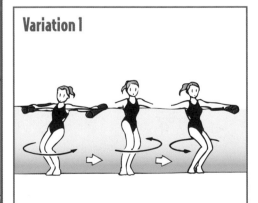

Hula-Hoop

Lay both hands on one aqua noodle beside you, bend your knees and twist your pelvis.

Variation 2

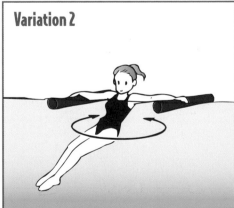

Buttocks

Lay both hands on one aqua noodle beside you. Do not touch the floor, turn your pelvis to the right and left and keep your legs stable. This is an advanced exercise. You can also bend your knees to modify the exercise.

Toning 4 – Turn and Shift your Weight

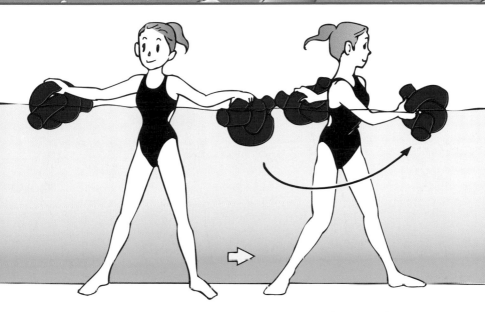

Shift your weight and turn your torso (Strengthening 1). This stretches your stomach and obliques and requires good coordination. The picture shows a person holding one knotted aqua noodle in each hand, pushing the aqua noodle with the right hand under the water, shifting the weight on the left leg and moving the aqua noodle to the left side. Have a sturdy stance.

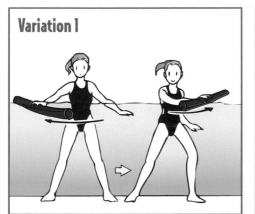

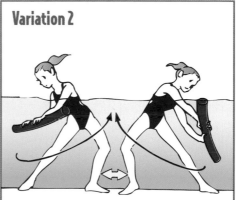

Arm-cross

Hold onto the aqua noodle with your right arm. Now move your extended arm from the left side over to the right side. While doing so, shift your weight on your left leg.

Scoop

Push the stick (a short aqua noodle) with both hands under water: arms should be extended, then scoop the aqua noodle to the other side. The buoyancy of the water is very high during this exercise.

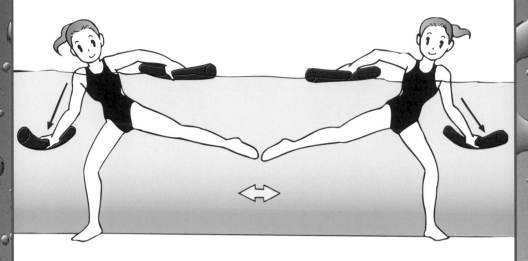

Tilt your torso side to side without turning it. Keep your torso sturdy. The picture shows a person pushing the aqua noodle in the water while rocking back and forth. While doing so, extend your other leg to the other side. A combination with shifting the weight side to side is possible. Keep your head upright (do not swing your head).

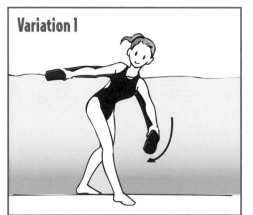

Variation 1

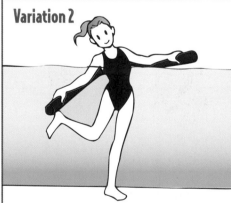

Variation 2

Bowling
Put the aqua noodle behind you and hold onto the ends. Now, push one end from the back down to the front. Watch out for your flank.

Touching your heel
Put the aqua noodle behind you and hold onto the ends. Now, bend your knee back toward your buttocks and push one end of the aqua noodle toward the heel of the same side. You do not have to touch your heel.

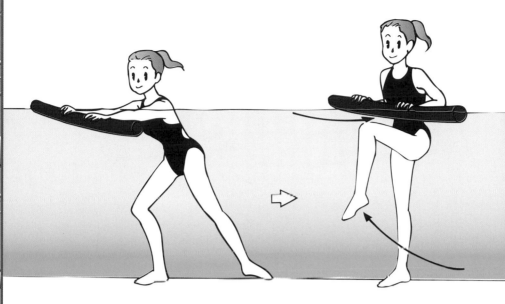

Hold onto the aqua noodle in front of you with both hands and pull it toward your torso. At the same time, pull your knee up (exhale). While doing so, tilt your body slightly to the front. You can also walk forward during this exercise. If you pull your knee up diagonally, you work your obliques.

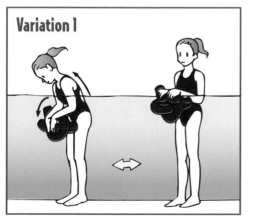

Variation 1

Bending your torso

Hold the knotted aqua noodle in front of your stomach. By tilting your body to the front you are pushing the aqua noodle under water (exhale). Then straighten your torso again. While doing so, pull your shoulders down.

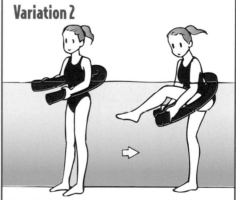

Variation 2

Under the knee

Put the aqua noodle behind you and hold onto the ends. Tilt your body forward and at the same time, pull one leg up. Now, bring the ends of the aqua noodle under your knee together. When straightening your back again, do not overextend.

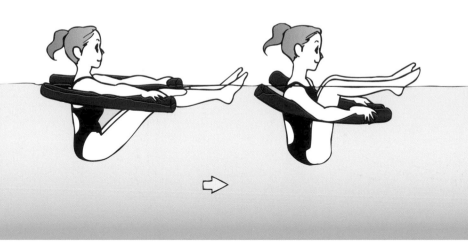

Lean each arm on one aqua noodle, bring both legs up and make the ends of the aqua noodles touch under your knees. While doing so, tilt your torso slightly forward. Do not swing. The aqua noodles do not necessarily have to touch.

Variation 1

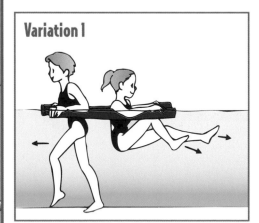

Leg press

Extend and flex your legs alternately and push the water with your heels away from you. Do not kick but press with your heels by flexing your toes. Do not swing so that you use your abdominal muscles and so that you are gentle on your hips.

Variation 2

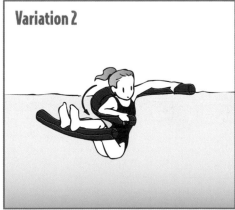

Turn

Lie on two aqua noodles, one under your arms holding tight to the ends and the other under your knees. Now, turn your torso to the left and right. (Not for rehabilitation).

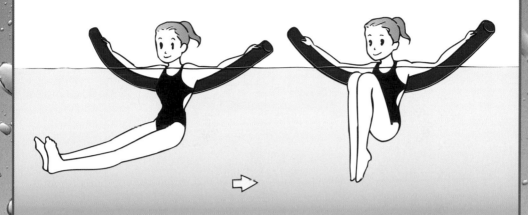

Put the aqua noodle under your arms. Your body is vertical, your extended legs are in a 90° angle to your torso. Now, bend your legs slowly toward your abdominal and then back in the extended position
Do not swing.
Variation: Parting the legs left and right alternately.

Variation 1

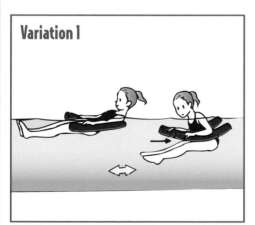

Variation 2

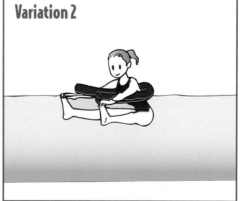

V-position
Put one aqua noodle under each arm. By tilting your pelvis back and down your torso changes from the horizontal into the vertical position. Keep your shoulders and your torso loose. This is an advanced exercise.

Grasping the toes
Your torso is in a vertical line, your legs are parted. Now, touch your toes with your hands. Variation: Alternate left and right. You do not necessarily have to touch your toes. Be careful of your balance.

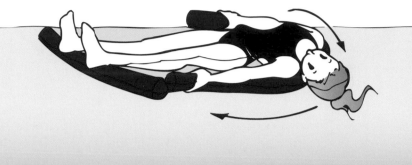

Lie backward on two aqua noodles, one under your arms and the other under your ankles. Now, tilt your torso to the left by moving your left hand toward your left foot. Do the same to the right side as far as your body allows you to go.

Variation 1

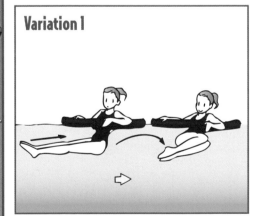

Crouch, turn, twist and extend
Your torso is in a vertical line, your legs are in a 90° angle to your torso. Now, pull your knees diagonally toward your shoulders. Move slowly and do not swing.

Variation 2

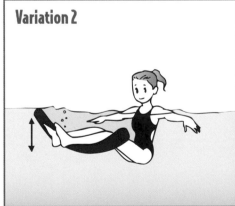

Press
Put the aqua noodle under your ankles, your legs are in a 90° angle to your torso and your arms are extended to your side for balance. Now, try to press your extended legs with the aqua noodle down against the resistance of the water. Do not swing. This is an advanced exercise. (Not suitable for people with back problems!).

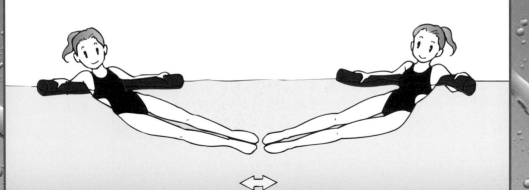

Lean backward on the aqua noodle. Extend your legs to the side. Now, bend your knees and extend your legs to the other side. Watch out for your balance.

Variation 1

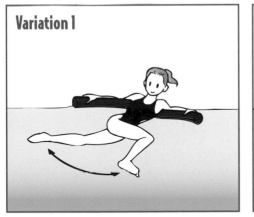

Variation 2

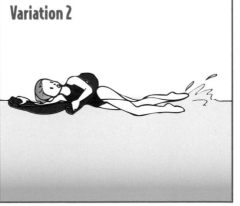

Straddle position (parting your legs)

Lean backward on the aqua noodle. Extend your legs to the right side. Then, bend your right knee over your extended left leg pulling it over to your left shoulder.

Swimming

Put the aqua noodle under your arms from the back and put your body in a horizontal line but facing your body to the front. Now, move your legs as if you were crawling. Find the best starting position on the aqua noodle for your balance.

Stretching · Coordination · Cardio Training

Toning

Fun & Play · Massage & Relaxation

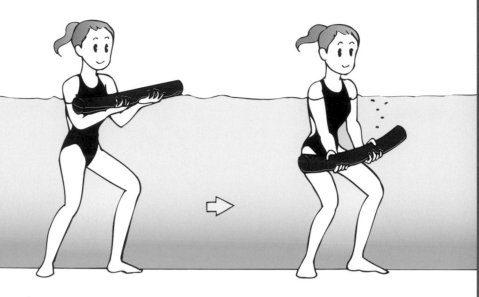

Grasp the aqua noodle from the bottom, extend and flex your arms. You can also use a stick (a short aqua noodle) for less resistance or you can also grasp the aqua noodle from the top.

Variation 1

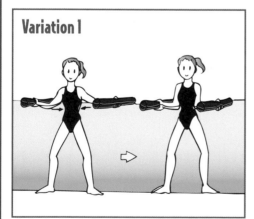

Variation 2

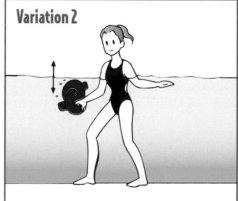

Grasp one short or knotted aqua noodle with each hand. Extend your arms. Now, bend your arms by moving your elbows toward your torso.

Push the knotted aqua noodle under the water as if you were dribbling a ball. Just a little pressure is enough.

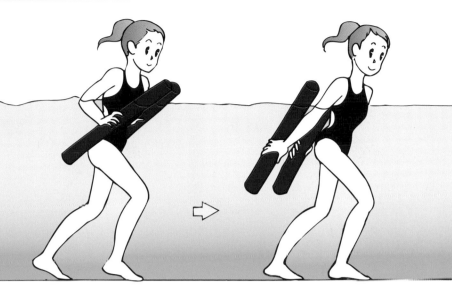

Hold onto one short aqua noodle (a stick) with each hand. Now, bend your elbows to the back, extending your arms. Only your forearm is moving, your upper arm stays stable. You can also extend your forearm alternately. When doing so, do not over-extend.

Variation 1

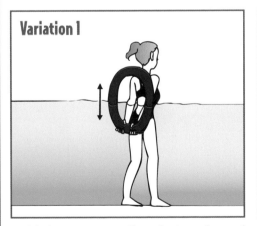

Hold the aqua noodle, which is formed like a ring, behind your back with extended arms. Now, move the aqua noodle up and down. Do not hyperextend. Keep your abdominal muscles connected.

Variation 2

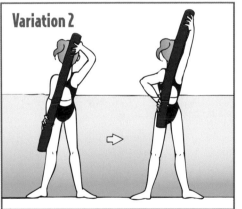

Hold the aqua noodle diagonally behind your back and move it up and down. Extend and flex your upper arm.

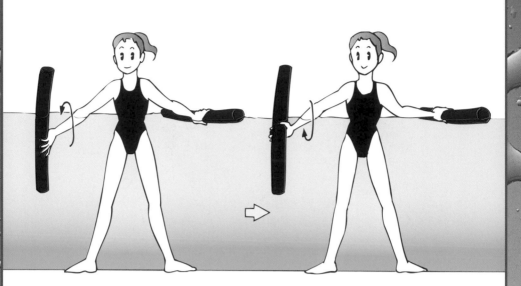

Place each hand on one aqua noodle. Now, turn your forearm under the water out and in. Your upper arm stays stable. If the resistance is too high then you can perform the exercise on the surface of the water. Perform the exercise either with both arms at the same time or alternately.

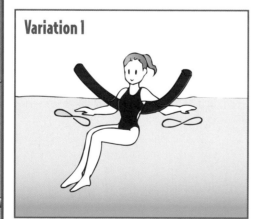

Variation 1

Squeeze the aqua noodle from the back under your arms. Keep your torso vertical and your legs bent in a sitting position without touching the floor. Now, draw the number eight with your hands. Your wrists should stay stable. Do not lock your elbows.

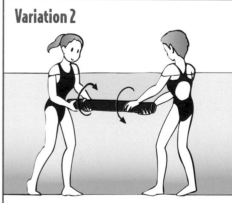

Variation 2

Two people face each other and hold onto the ends of one aqua noodle with both hands. Now, turn the aqua noodle in the opposite direction. Perform this slowly. Keep the forearms prone and supine.

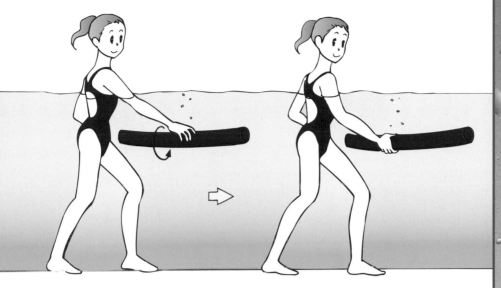

Hold onto the aqua noodle with one hand and turn your wrist in and out. This exercise can be performed under water or on the surface of the water, each time very slowly.

Variation 1

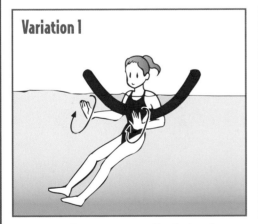

Squeeze the aqua noodle behind your back under your arms. Twist your wrist. Keep your fingers spread or together (scoop or fan your hands).

Variation 2

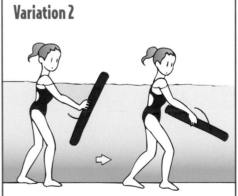

Hold the aqua noodle with one hand in a vertical line underwater or on the surface of the water.

Stretching · Coordination · Cardio Training · Toning · Fun & Play · Massage & Relaxation

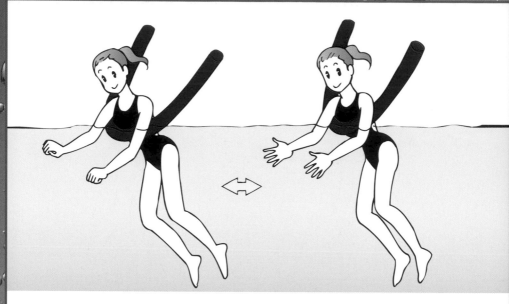

Squeeze the aqua noodle under your arms in front of you. Now, squeeze your fingers together and then spread them apart. Variation: Squeeze tightly, spread wide, move one finger at a time.

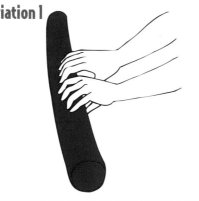

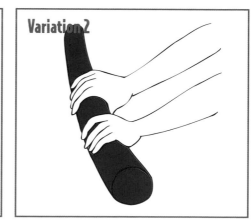

Variation 1

Variation 2

Pinching

Pinch the aqua noodle with your fingers together. The aqua noodle is under or on the surface of the water. This exercise is suitable for therapy.

Grabbing

Grasp the aqua noodle tightly using your entire palm. The aqua noodle is under or on the surface of the water. This exercise is suitable for therapy.

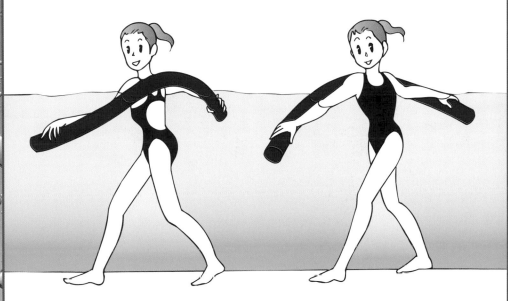

Put the aqua noodle behind you and grasp the two ends. Now, move your arms as if you were crawling. The aqua noodle can be on the surface of the water. You can also move your arms as if you were swimming on your back.

Variation 1

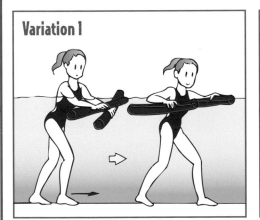

Hold one aqua noodle in each hand and move your arms as if you were crawling. The aqua noodle can be on the surface of the water. Variation: Change the direction of the arms, e.g. cross the arms.

Variation 2

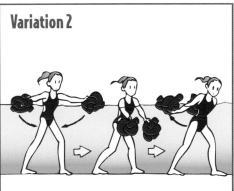

Butterfly-swimming
Hold one knotted aqua noodle in each hand and move your arms as if you were doing the butterfly in swimming. Push the aqua noodle only as far as necessary.

Stretching · Coordination · Cardio Training

Toning

Fun & Play · Massage & Relaxation

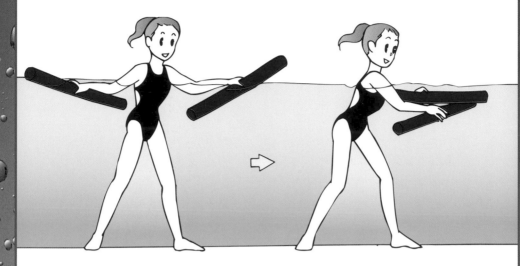

Grasp one short aqua noodle (a stick) with each hand. Now, move the arms as if you were playing tennis. Keep the aqua noodle in a vertical or horizontal line like a backhand or a forehand movement in tennis.

Variation 1

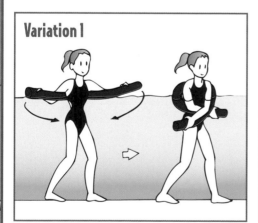

Squeeze the aqua noodle under your arms behind your back. Now press the ends in front of you together with slightly extended arms.

Variation 2

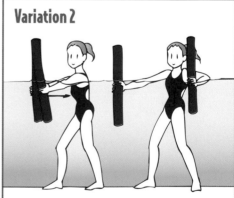

Hold one aqua noodle in each hand in a vertical line in front of you. Now, move your arms as if you were shooting a bow and arrow.

Hold one aqua noodle in a vertical line in front of your body with both hands. Now pull the aqua noodle to the right and left. Half of the aqua noodle is under the water. For an advanced exercise, push the whole aqua noodle under water.

Variation 1

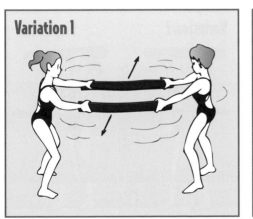

Two people are facing each other and holding onto two aqua noodles with extended arms, moving the aqua noodles symmetrically out and in.

Variation 2

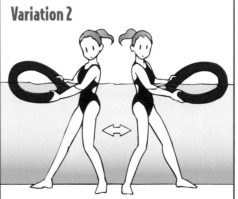

Pull the aqua noodle, which is formed like a ring, through the water, to the left and right.
Variation: Change the resistance by changing the angle of the aqua noodle.

Stretching ○ Coordination ○ Cardio Training

Toning

Fun & Play ○ Massage & Relaxation

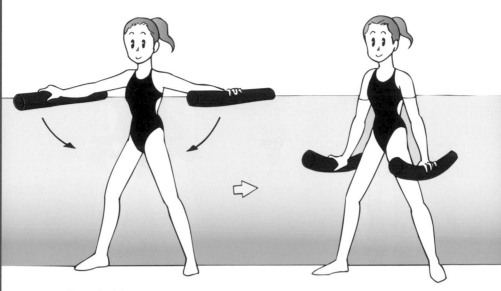

Part your legs, hold one aqua noodle on each side. Now, push your extended arms down towards your thighs. Variation: Perform the exercise in front of your body.

Variation 1

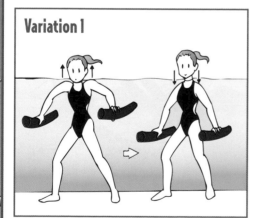

Part your legs, hold one aqua noodle on each side and keep your arms extended. Now, pull your shoulders up and back down.

Variation 2

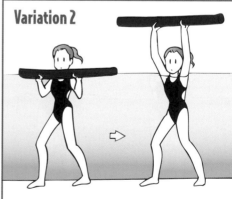

Lift

Hold the aqua noodle in a horizontal line with both hands in front of your body. Now, lift your hands up and down. You can perform this exercise in a standing or supine position.

Stretching

Coordination

Toning

Fun & Play

Massage & Relaxation

Toning 22 – Hold up

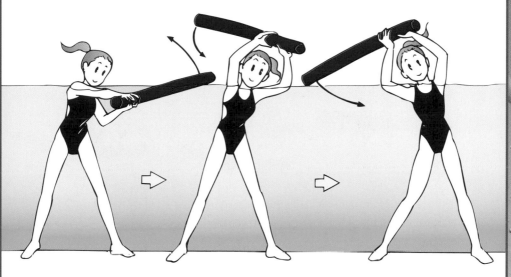

Hold the aqua noodle with both hands up in the air and move it behind your head as if you were throwing a ball. Keep your shoulders under water. You can also perform this exercise with one hand.

Variation 1

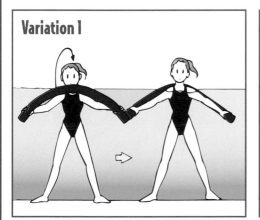

Grasp the ends of the aqua noodle with your hands and lift it up over your head behind your back. If this is too hard, you can just move the aqua noodle up and down in front of your body.

Variation 2

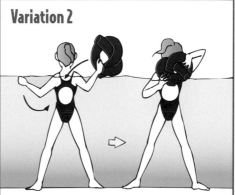

Hold the knotted aqua noodle in one hand. Then, take the aqua noodle from one hand in the other hand by putting your elbow over your shoulder and taking the aqua noodle in your other hand by putting your other hand up toward your shoulder blade.

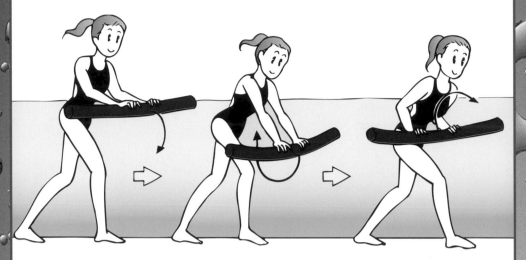

Grasp the aqua noodle with both hands and hold it in front of you in a horizontal line. Then, make a big circle keeping the aqua noodle horizontal. Variation: Make the circles smaller, bigger or change directions. You can also perform the exercise within a group or with a partner.

Variation 1

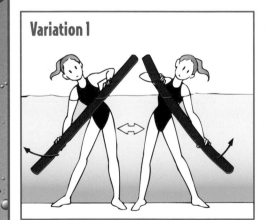

Grasp the aqua noodle with both hands and hold it in front of you in a horizontal line. Then, move it as if you were paddling. Variation: You can also perform the exercise backward.

Variation 2

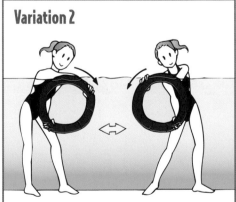

Turn the knotted aqua noodle around as if you were driving. The aqua noodle does not necessarily have to be in the water. Watch out that you do not strain your shoulder joint.

Stretching · Coordination · Toning · Fun & Play · Message & Relaxation

Grasp the aqua noodle with both hands and hold it in front of you in a horizontal line. Now, move the aqua noodle from side to side. You can also use your legs. Beginners should use a short aqua noodle (a stick).

Variation 1

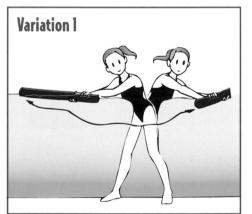

Snake

Grasp one end of the aqua noodle with both hands and move like a snake. The exercise is not only for your arms but also for your torso and flank.

Variation 2

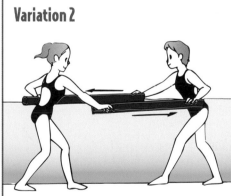

Sawing

Two people facing each other hold the ends of two aqua noodles in their hands. Now, pull back and forth. Do not use too much force.

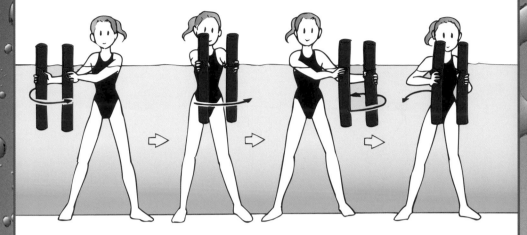

Grasp two aqua noodles and hold them in a vertical line in front of you. Then, make circles as if you were stirring. Variation: Grasp the aqua noodle higher or lower, turn right and left alternately, faster and slower or use shorter aqua noodles.

Variation 1

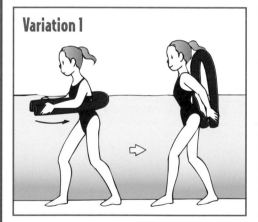

Grasp the aqua noodle, keeping it behind your back. Then, bring the ends together either in front of you or behind you. You can also combine this exercise with adjusting your weight from one leg to the other.

Variation 2

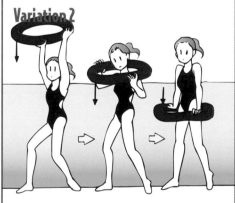

Hold the aqua noodle formed like a ring, up in the air keeping your shoulders under water. Then, bring the aqua noodle down along your body. If this exercise is too hard, stop at shoulder level.

Two people face each other holding onto the ends of one aqua noodle that makes a big circle while keeping the aqua noodle in a horizontal line. Keep your elbows and wrist unlocked.

Toning

Variation 1

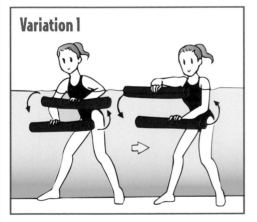

Variation 2

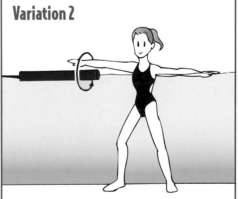

Grasp one aqua noodle in each hand, keep both in front of you, and draw circles while keeping the aqua noodles in a horizontal line. You can also perform this exercise with a short aqua noodle (a stick).

Keep your shoulders under water, the aqua noodle is on the surface of the water, your arms are extended to your sides. Now, make a circle with your forearm around the aqua noodle. This exercise is also suitable for therapy.

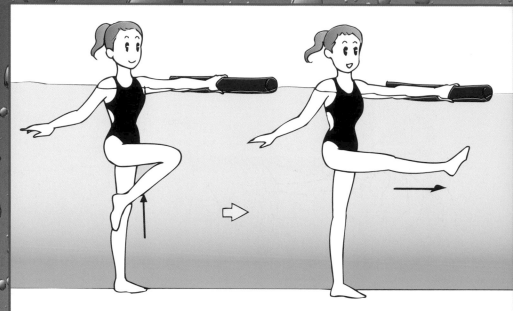

Hold onto the aqua noodle sideways, parallel to the floor. Bend one knee up in a 90° angle to your torso and slowly extend and then bend your leg again. Variation: Change directions.

Variation 1

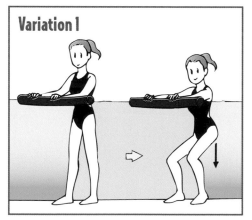

Squat and come back up. You can leave your legs apart or bring them together. Keep your foot on the floor. When pushing the aqua noodle under water, the buoyancy of the water increases.

Variation 2

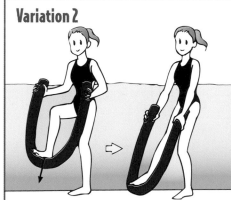

Leg-press
Put your foot on the aqua noodle and extend your leg toward the floor. Keep an eye on your balance. To intensify the exercise let go of the aqua noodle.

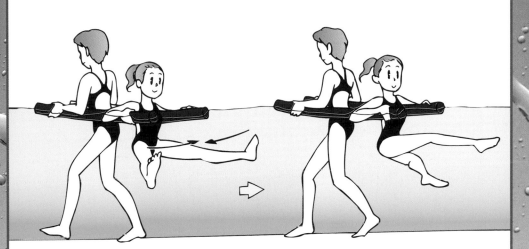

Two people stand back to back and hold onto two aqua noodles. One person bends the legs in a 90° angle to the torso and opens and closes the legs. Keeping your torso straight up, you are working your back muscles. The other person moves forward at the same time.

Variation 1

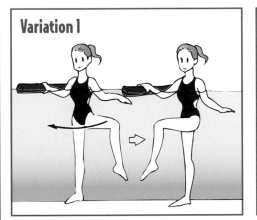

Hold onto one aqua noodle on the side and bend one knee up in a 90° angle to your torso. Now, move your knee in and out.

Variation 2

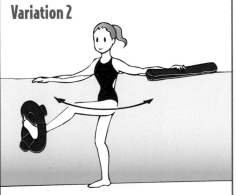

Hold onto one aqua noodle on the side and put a knotted aqua noodle around your foot. Now turn your leg from your hip out and in. The buoyancy is very high. That is why you have to be careful not to overexert the hip.

Stretching · Coordination · Cardio Training

Toning

Fun & Play · Massage & Relaxation

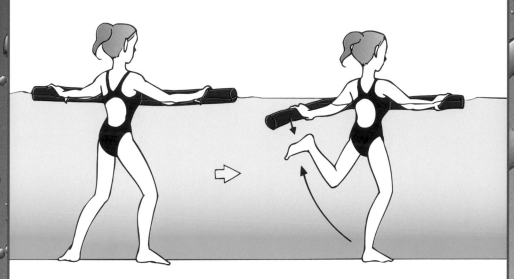

Hold onto one aqua noodle and stand sturdy. Pull your heel toward your buttocks. Do not overextend.

Variation 1

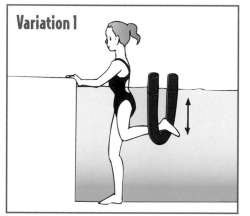

Face the edge of the pool and hold onto the side. Put the aqua noodle around your ankle and move your foot up and down. Make small moves due to the high buoyancy of the water.

Variation 2

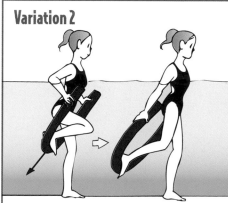

Hold onto the aqua noodle with both hands, put your foot on the aqua noodle and extend your leg to the back. Do not swing or overextend your back, otherwise it can be too much of a strain on your hip.

Stretching

Coordination

Fun & Play

Massage & Relaxation

Toning

Toning 30 – Toes and Heels

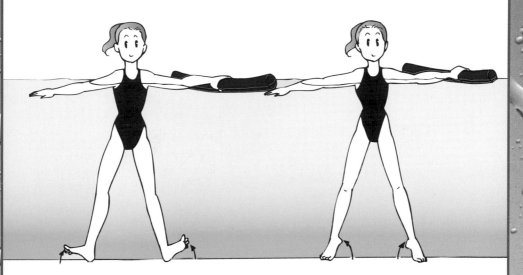

Hold onto the aqua noodle, stand with your legs apart, knees facing outwards while balancing and alternating on your heels and toes. Stay on the same spot or move your legs farther apart, like a split. Perform this exercise with caution because cramps may occur.

Variation 1

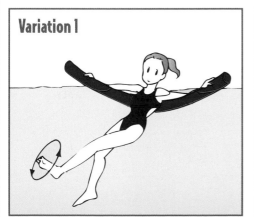

Lie on your back on the aqua noodle circling your ankles in and out or drawing the number eight with your toes.

Variation 2

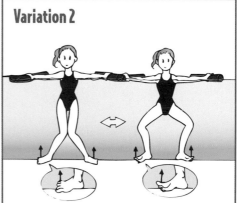

Hold onto one aqua noodle on each side. Now, turn your feet in and out alternately while keeping your knees bent. If you have knee or ankle-joint problems perform this exercise with caution.

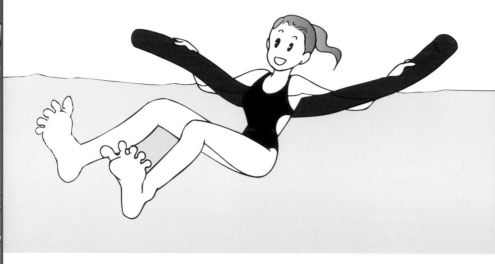

Spread your toes and relax again. You can perform this exercise while lying on the aqua noodle on your back or while being in a standing position. This exercise is also suitable for therapy.

Variation 1

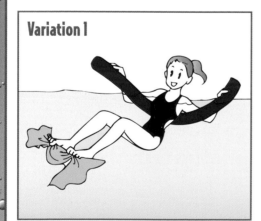

Lie on your back on the aqua noodle and grab, for example, a bath cap with your toes. This is a suitable workout for your toes.

Variation 2

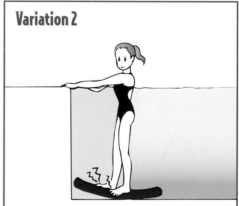

Stand on the aqua noodle with both feet. You can also perform this exercise with short aqua noodles. This is suitable for therapy. This exercise is good to desensitize the soles of your feet.

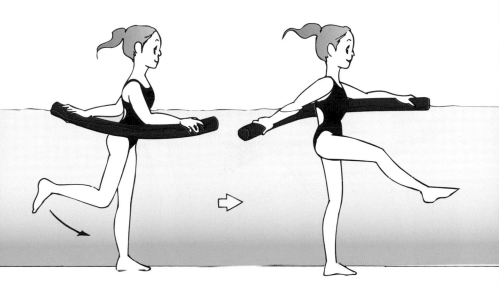

Hold the aqua noodle behind your back, bend one leg to the back and then kick it to the front as if you were playing soccer. Keep your torso straight up. Do not swing your hips or overextend your back.

Variation 1

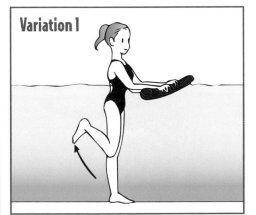

Hold onto one aqua noodle with both hands. Then, pull your heels toward your buttocks alternately. Do not swing your hips or overextend your back.

Variation 2

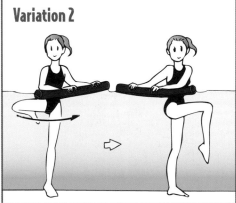

Hold onto one aqua noodle with both hands, bend your knee to the side and then bring your leg to the front crossing your extended leg with your shin as if you were doing karate.

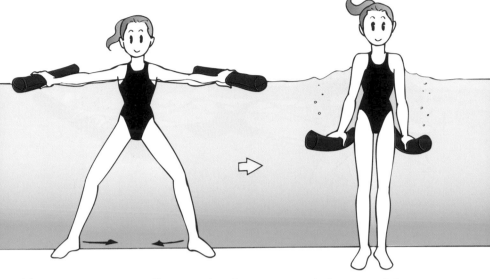

Hold onto one aqua noodle on each side. Your extended arms stabilize your stance, your legs are apart. Now, jump up bringing your legs together and your extended arms toward your torso. You can also perform this exercise without using your arms.

Variation 1

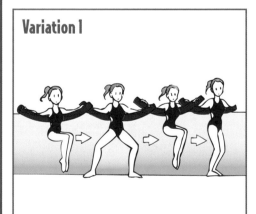

Lie down backward on the aqua noodle bending your knees and then bringing them back to the floor in a squat position. Bend your knees again, but this time bring your legs together to the floor. This exercise works your abdominal muscles and your buttocks.

Variation 2

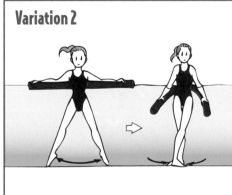

Put the aqua noodle behind you and hold onto it keeping your legs apart. Then, cross your legs. You can also cross your arms. This intensifies the exercise.

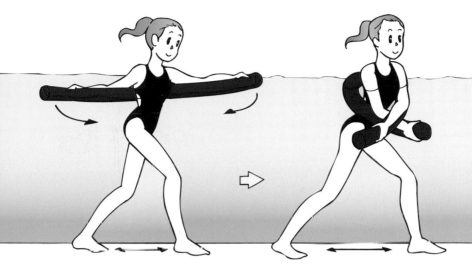

Put the aqua noodle behind you and hold on to it. Your legs are in a lunge position alternating your left and right leg in the air. Variation: With or without arms, increase the speed. The picture shows the exercise with synchronized arms.

Variation 1

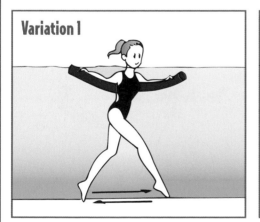

Hold the aqua noodle behind your back, keeping your shoulders under water. Bring your left and right leg alternately back and forth while keeping contact with the floor with your toes. Keep your torso sturdy, which means no up and down movement.

Variation 2

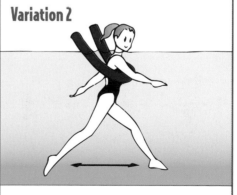

Deep water: Lean on the aqua noodle while performing the same exercise as in Variation 1. It is not easy to keep your balance. Use your arms for balance.

Stretching · Coordination · Cardio Training · Toning · Fun & Play · Massage & Relaxation

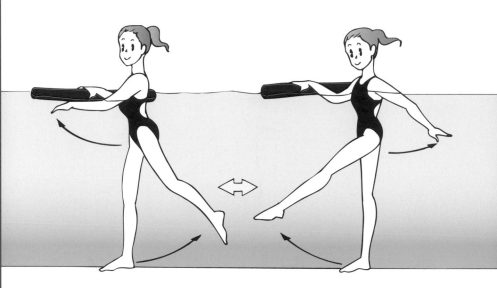

Hold onto the aqua noodle on the side while bringing one extended leg back and forth but not too far to the back because you will risk hyperextension. Use your arms for balance.

Variation 1

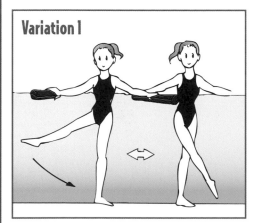

Hold onto the aqua noodle on the side. Stand sturdy on one leg while lifting the other to the left and to the right. Alternate sides. Keep your back straight and watch out that you do not strain your hip.

Variation 2

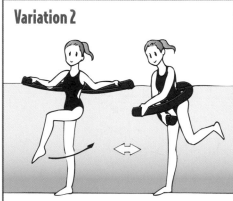

Hold onto the aqua noodle behind you, bend your knee up, then bring it to the back and to the front. This exercise is for beginners.

Stretching

Coordination

Cardio Training

Toning

Fun & Play

Massage & Relaxation

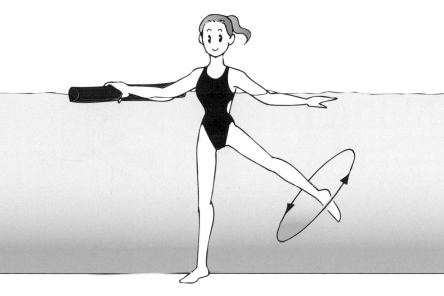

Extend one leg and circle it or draw a number. Variation: Move your torso, with or without the aqua noodle for support.

Variation 1

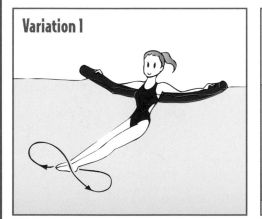

Lie backward on the aqua noodle and draw the number eight with your legs. This works the flexibility in your hip joint.

Variation 2

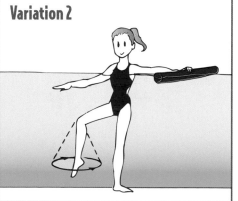

Hold onto the aqua noodle next to you, bend one knee up and circle your lower leg. Variation: Make bigger/smaller circles, change direction, increase or decrease speed.

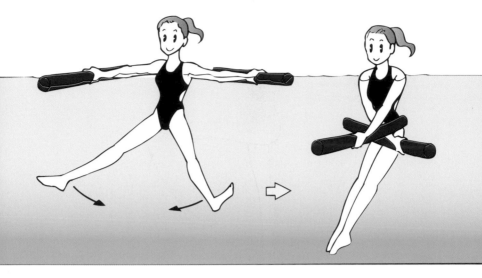

Hold onto one aqua noodle on each side while opening and closing your legs. Use your arms at the same time as the picture shows. This exercise provides no stability and therefore is an advanced one. If you keep an angle of 90° between your legs and your torso, you work your abdominal muscles harder.

Variation 1

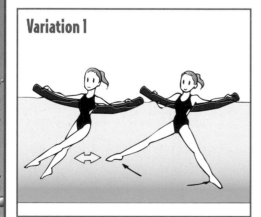

Variation 2

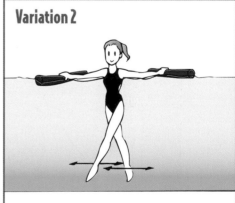

Lie backward on the aqua noodle and cross your legs, keeping them extended. You can keep the 90° angle to make it harder or keep your body in one line to make it easier.

Deep water: Hold onto one aqua noodle on each side keeping your body in a vertical line. Now, cross your legs. This exercise improves your posture.

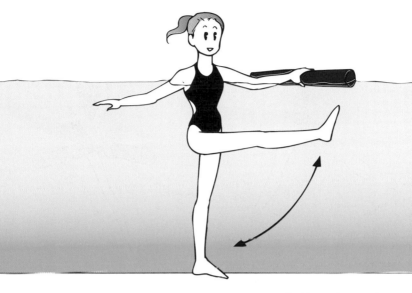

Grasp one aqua noodle on the side and lift your extended leg. This works your hip and thigh. Perform this exercise slowly and do not swing. The picture shows a person lifting the leg to the front. Variation: Lift one knee diagonally up and turn your torso.

Variation 1

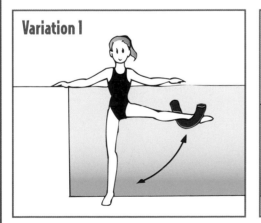

Lay one leg on the aqua noodle next to you moving it up and down. Use a short aqua noodle due to the high buoyancy of the water, which makes the exercise more intense.

Variation 2

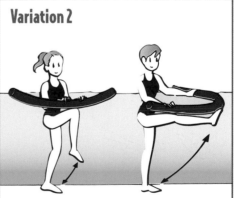

Hold one aqua noodle in front of you in a horizontal line. Now, pull your knee or your toes toward the aqua noodle. You can also put the aqua noodle behind you.

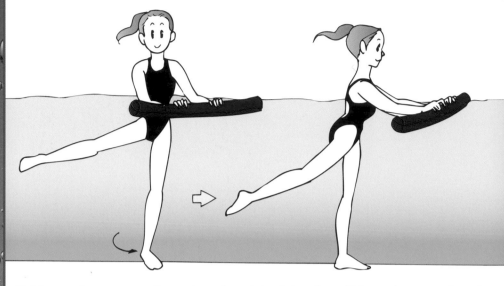

Hold onto the aqua noodle on the side with both hands and lift one leg up to the other side. Jump up with your other leg and turn at the same time. This exercise works your buttocks, torso and hip joint. The picture shows a 90° turn of the torso.

Variation 1

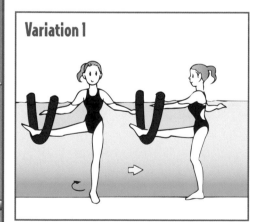

Put your lifted leg on the aqua noodle and jump with your other leg and turn. This advanced exercise stretches and strengthens your body due to the high buoyancy of the water.

Variation 2

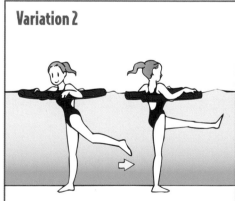

Hold onto one aqua noodle on each side and lift one leg back. Make a 180° turn so your leg is now in front of you. You can either take the aqua noodle with you or just jump and land on it again.

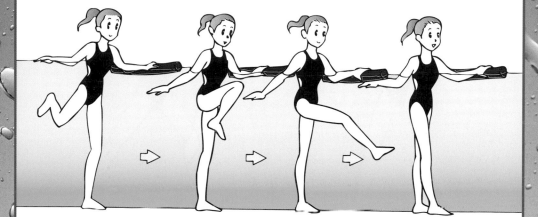

Improving the flexibility of your hip joint: Bend your leg to the back and then extend it to the front. The picture shows a typical exercise, that athletes perform on land. Do not swing. Use the aqua noodle for support.

Variation 1

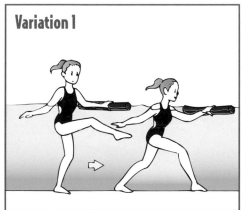

Make big steps moving forward. Do not overextend your back when landing. Use the aqua noodle for support on your side.

Variation 2

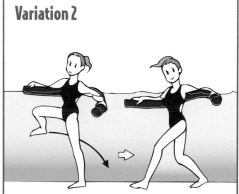

Hold the aqua noodle behind you and make big steps, bending your leg diagonally to the back walking backward. Do not overextend your back.

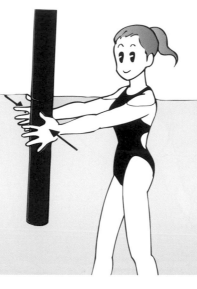

Produce an isometric contraction by squeezing the aqua noodle together with your hands or fingers from the left and right. Hold it for 20 seconds, continue breathing and keep your other body parts loose.

Variation 1

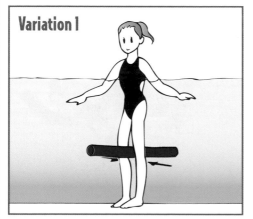

Put the aqua noodle between your thighs and squeeze them together. You can also try and move forward.

Variation 2

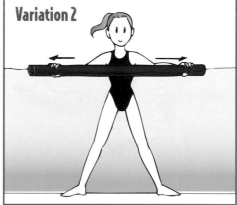

Keep your arms bent and pull the aqua noodle apart and hold it there. Keep an eye on your shoulders and your chest.

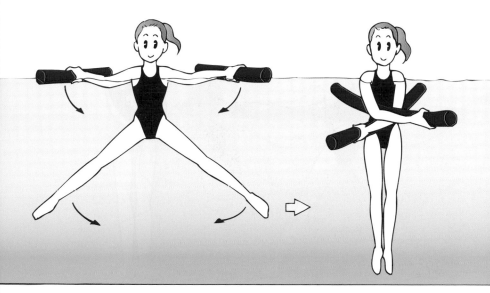

Jumping Jack

Hold on to one aqua noodle on each side. Keep arms and legs extended and wide apart and then bring them back together. Keep your entire body stable.

Variation 1

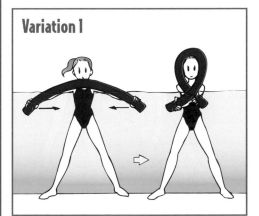

Grasp the ends of the aqua noodle, keeping your arms extended. Now, cross your arms in front of you forming a ring with the aqua noodle and hold it there.

Variation 2

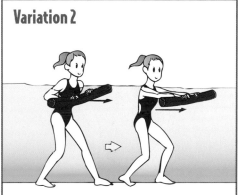

Grasp the aqua noodle in front of you. The aqua noodle is kept in a horizontal line. Now, pull the aqua noodle toward your body and then push it away. This exercises your chest. Do this a few times to learn the exercise.

Stretching · Coordination · Cardio Training

Toning

Fun & Play · Massage & Relaxation

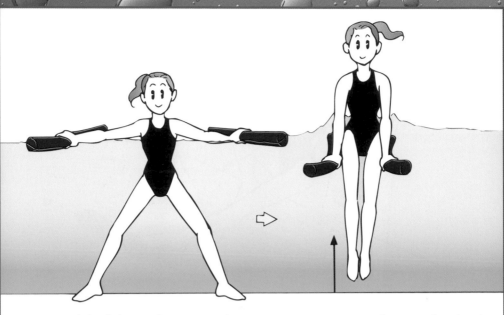

Jump up with both legs or hop on one leg. Lean on one aqua noodle on each side. The picture shows a person with the legs apart jumping up and closing the legs at the same time.

Variation 1

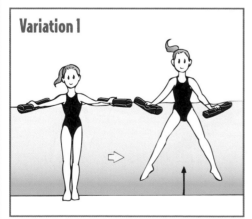

Same starting position: now keep your legs closed. Jump up and open your legs. Come back down, either with your legs apart or together.

Variation 2

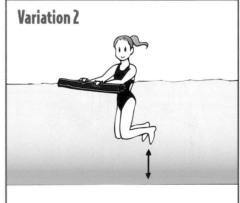

Grasp the aqua noodle, which is in front of you. Keep it in a horizontal line. Now, bend both knees toward your buttocks at the same time. Do not overextend.

Stretching
Coordination
Cardio Training
Toning
Fun & Play
Massage & Relaxation

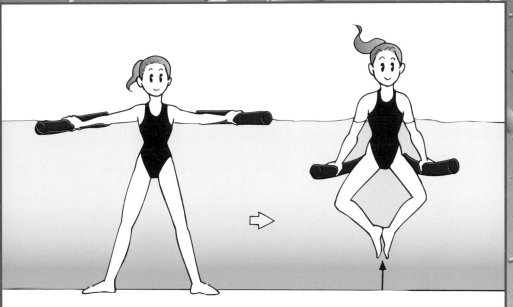

Put one aqua noodle on each of your side and hold onto it, keeping your legs apart. Now, jump up and make your feet touch. Repeat this exercise.

Variation 1

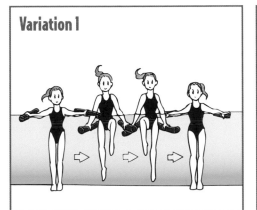

Same starting position: Jump up and pull your knees up alternately.

Variation 2

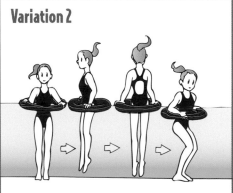

Put the aqua noodle, which is formed like a ring, around your body and jump up. At the same time, turn around on your own axis (90° or 180°). When you turn, you can hold onto the aqua noodle or let go.

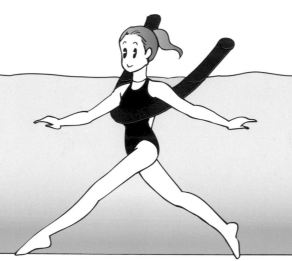

Your legs are in a lunge and your shoulders are under water. Squeeze the aqua noodle under your arms in the front. The picture shows long water specific strides for best effects. The upper body should stay vertical. Keep your legs together at the end of the exercise.

Variation 1

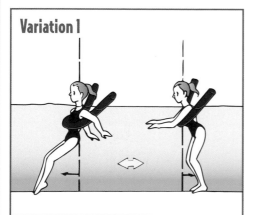

Variation 2

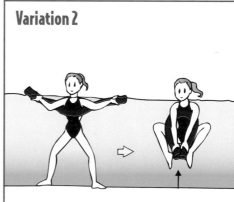

Same starting position: Your torso stays in a vertical line. Now, jump with both legs to the front or to the back without moving your torso.

Squeeze the aqua noodle under your arms from the front and hold on tightly to the ends. Now, bend both knees out. At the same time, your heels should touch the ends of the aqua noodle. Alternate left and right or touch both at the same time.

Stretching

Coordination

Toning

Fun & Play

Massage & Relaxation

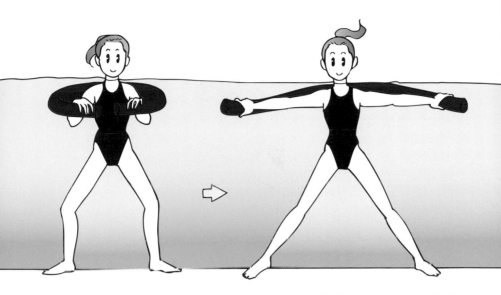

Keep your legs apart and your shoulders under water. Hold the aqua noodle behind your shoulder blades. Now, part your legs and close them again. There are many more movements possible in the water than on land, e.g. you can part your legs much wider so that the strain on your hips and legs is released. Bring your legs back together keeping contact with the floor.

Variation 1

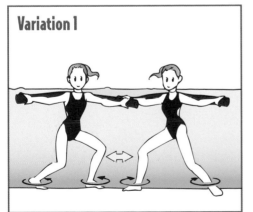

Your legs are apart, keep your torso, head and arms stable. Turn your hips in and out by turning your heels in and out.

Variation 2

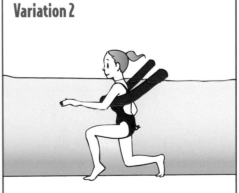

Squeeze the aqua noodle under your arms from the front. Now, move forward with your knees bent. Variation: Walk backward.

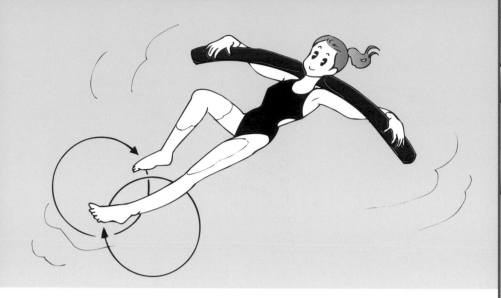

Lie in a supine position with your head on the aqua noodle and move your legs as if you were riding a bike. Variation: Lie in a prone position, on the side, etc.

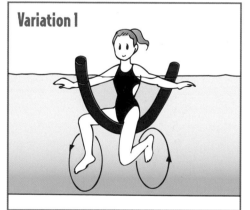

Variation 1

Sit on the aqua noodle. Beginners can hold onto the edge of the pool. Move your legs as if you were riding a bike and use your arms for balance.

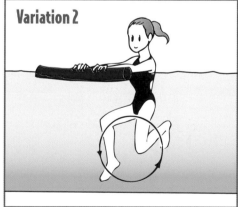

Variation 2

Hold onto the aqua noodle. In a standing position, move one leg as if you were riding a bike. Alternate sides.

Toning 54 – Dynamic Stabilization

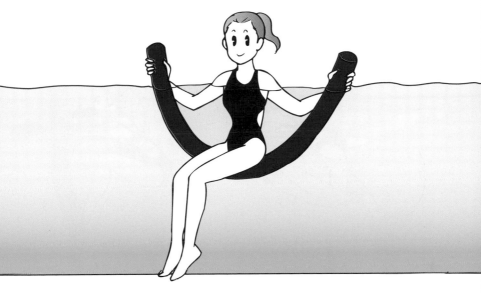

Sit on the aqua noodle and hold onto the ends next to you (or not). Move your pelvis around. Try to sit on the aqua noodle for a longer period of time. You can also touch the floor with your toes or your feet for balance. This exercise trains the "balance" of the upper body.

Variation 1

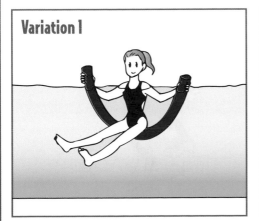

Same starting position: Now, try to keep your balance with extended legs. This is a more advanced exercise.

Variation 2

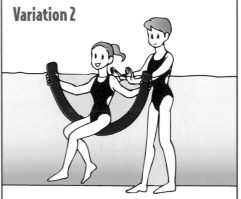

Same starting position: Another person tries to bring the partner out of balance by producing waves. The person on the aqua noodle has to try and work against the resistance.

FUN & PLAY

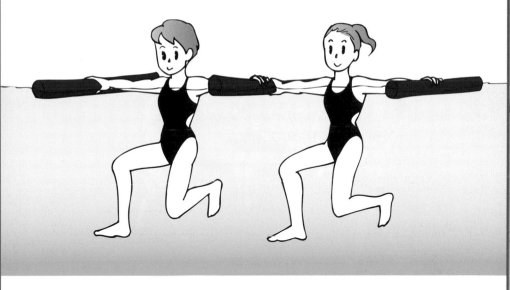

This exercise is good for communication and to enjoy the movement in the water. Several different creative group formations are possible. The picture shows two people riding a bike together. Form a group or a line while riding the bike and hold on to the aqua noodles next to you.

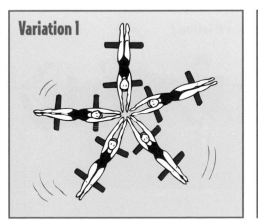

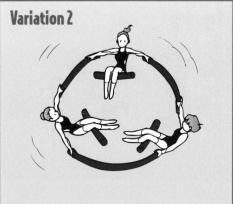

Variation 1

The star formation
This exercise is also possible with aqua noodles formed like a ring.

Variation 2

Run in a circle
Left or right, everybody or just every other person.

Stretching · Coordination · Cardio Training · Toning · **Fun & Play** · Massage & Relaxation

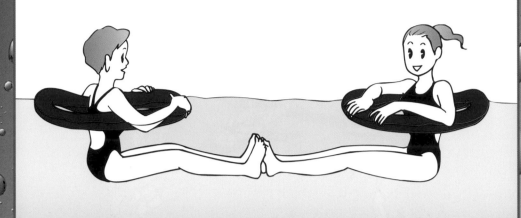

There are several possibilities. Choose safe exercises. The picture shows an exercise with communicating feet. The arms are leaned on the aqua noodle formed like a ring, the legs are extended to the front and the sole of the feet of the two people touch each other.

Variation 1

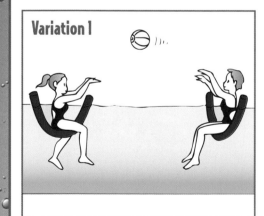

Two people sit on the aqua noodle and play ball.

Variation 2

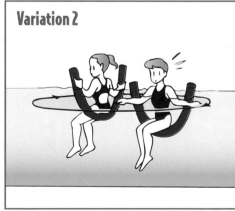

Finger game
Two people each sit on the aqua noodle, move their hands and fingers and turn on their own axis. You can also race against each other.

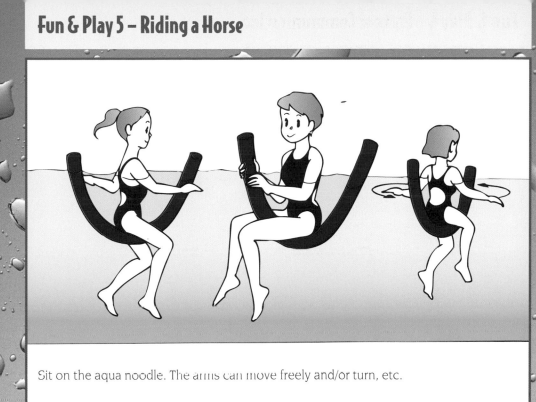

Sit on the aqua noodle. The arms can move freely and/or turn, etc.

Variation 1

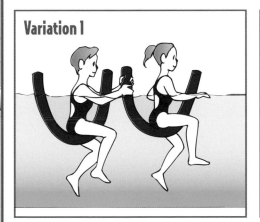

Variation 2

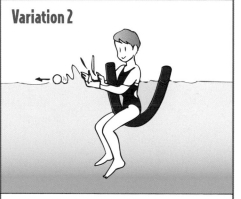

Ride behind each other. Each sits on the aqua noodle. The one in the back grasps the end of the aqua noodle in front of him. Form a line and move forward.

Sit on the aqua noodle and produce waves making the ball float away.

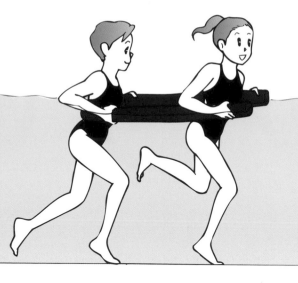

Two people hold two aqua noodles next to them. The one in the front holds it at flank height and the one in the back grasps the ends. Now, the two people should move forward.

Variation 1

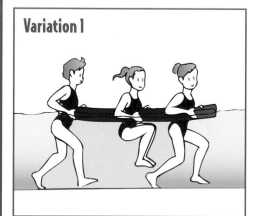

Variation 2

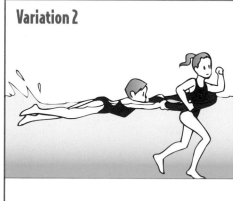

The train with three people: Same starting position. The one in the front and the one on the back jog forward. The person in the middle can hang loose.

Two people: One runs forward with the aqua noodle around the waistline. The one in the back grasps the ends of the aqua noodle, lies in a prone position and can also move the legs.

Fun & Play 7 – Basketball

A lot more equipment can be combined with the aqua noodle. The possibilities are endless. Use safe equipment. The picture shows two people playing basketball. Throw the ball in the net (an aqua noodle formed like a ring). You can vary the height of the net.

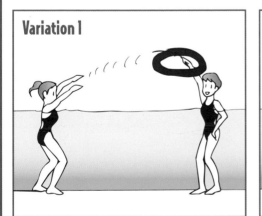

Variation 1

Throw the aqua noodle formed like a ring toward your partner. Your partner should extend his arms over his head.

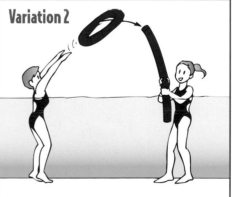

Variation 2

Try to throw the aqua noodle formed like a ring around another aqua noodle, which is kept in a vertical line. The partner can also move the aqua noodle around.

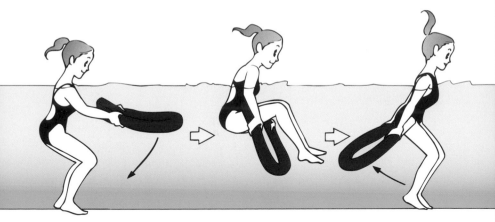

Jumping rope

Grasp the ends of the aqua noodle in front of you and jump over the rope keeping your legs together. Jumping over the rope with only one leg and then the other makes it easier.

Variation 1

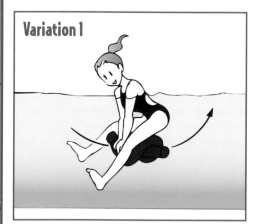

Jump over a floating, knotted aqua noodle with your legs apart. The beginner can push the aqua noodle down and move it through the legs.

Variation 2

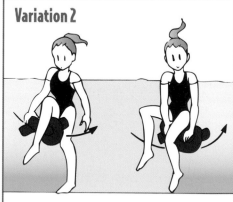

Push the knotted aqua noodle under your thighs. Advanced exercise: Bend both knees and push the knotted aqua noodle under them.

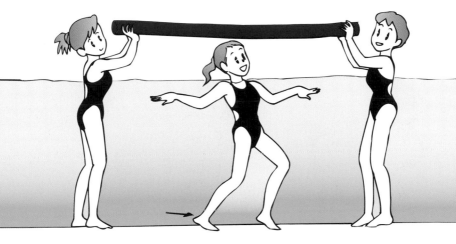

Two people hold the aqua noodle over the water. The third person walks under the aqua noodle. Bring the aqua noodle down with each pass underneath. Do not overextend.

Variation 1

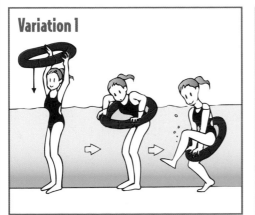

Walk through the aqua noodle formed like a ring. Begin with your head and work yourself down to your feet or start the other way.

Variation 2

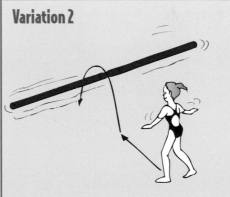

Form a long line with a couple of aqua noodles. Now try to jump over them. Vary the rules of the game: Use your hands, keep your legs together, jump over it with one leg and then the other.

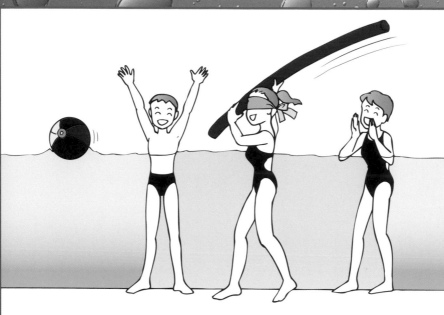

A person has to try to find a ball with her eyes blindfolded. The person has an aqua noodle in her hands and has to hit the ball. The others have to give the person clues.

Variation 1

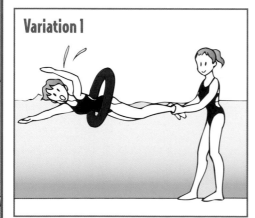

Variation 2

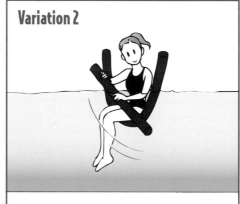

Put the aqua noodle formed like a ring around your waistline. Lie in a prone position and move your arms as if you were crawling. The partner holds the feet of the person crawling. This is an advanced exercise.

Sit on the aqua noodle and move your arms as if you were paddling with a short aqua noodle in your hands. Keep an eye on your balance.

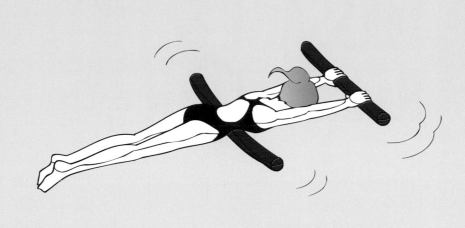

Lie in a prone position with your head under water. This exercise is to get used to the water or as a game for advanced level. The picture shows a person laying on two aqua noodles, one under the stomach and the other in the hands. Keep your arms extended over your head.

Variation 1

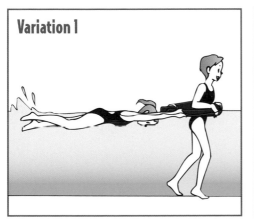

One person pulls another through the water. This trains the breathing system when crawling.

Variation 2

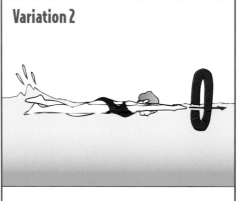

Try to swim through the aqua noodle formed like a ring. Lie in a prone position, move your legs as if you were crawling and extend your arms over your head.

MASSAGE & RELAXATION

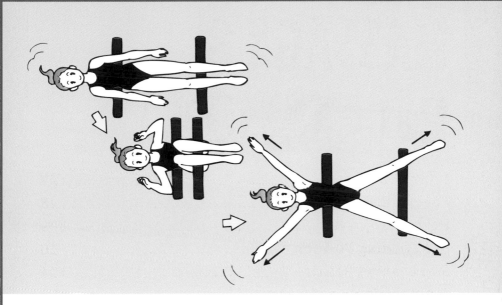

Lie on two aqua noodles in a supine position, one under your chest and the other under your knees. Stretch your body. The strain of gravity is lower in a horizontal position than in a vertical position (this is a therapeutic advantage). Extend your arms and legs forming an X. Now, bend your knees toward your stomach and bring your arms towards your head.

Variation 1

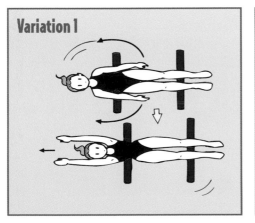

Arms
Same starting position: Extend your arms next to your ears and then back. In case you have shoulder problems, extend just as far as your body allows you.

Variation 2

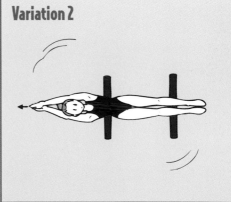

Shoulders
Same starting position: Your hands are clasped together and your arms are extended next to your head. Now, push your arms up keeping your arms in the extension of your vertebrae .

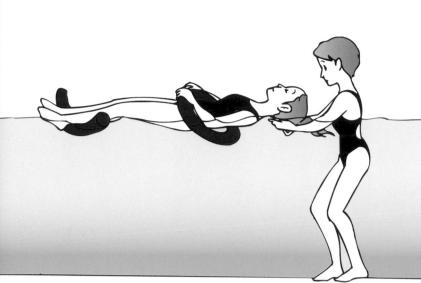

Lie on two aqua noodles in a supine position. One aqua noodle is under your ankles and the other one formed like a ring is around your torso. The partner is behind the head of the one floating in the water. This exercise is for massage and communication: The picture shows a massage for your torso, head, shoulders and back. Massage with your hands and find the spots with the most tension with your thumbs. The one receiving the massage should relax and keep breathing.

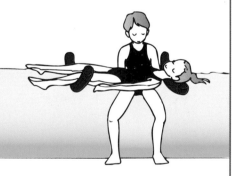

Variation 1

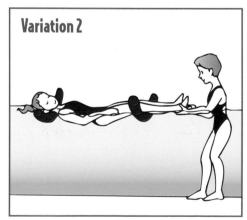

Variation 2

Stomach

Lie on two aqua noodles in a supine position, one under your knees and the other under your neck. The partner stands next to the person floating. Now slightly push the stomach and shake it.

Legs and feet

Same starting position: The second person is standing at the feet of the one lying down. Now, massage the feet and lower legs.

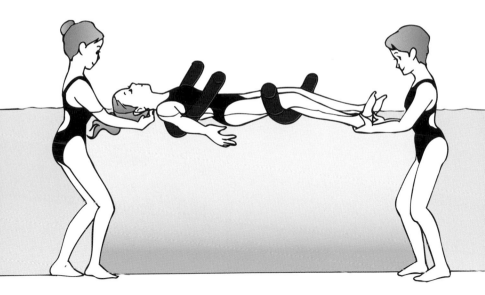

Lie on two aqua noodles in a supine position, one under your arms, the other under your knees. Now, the person lying down is getting a massage from the two people. One person massages the head, neck and shoulders, the other one massages the toes and the sole of the feet. The one lying down should relax.

Variation 1

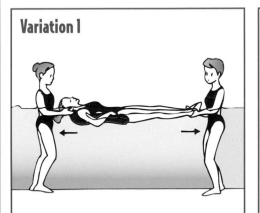

Extension

Same starting position: One person holds onto the other person´s head, the other person holds onto the feet. Now, they pull gently.

Variation 2

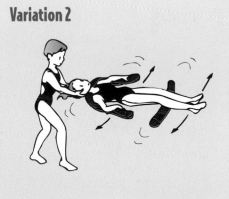

Rocking chair

Same starting position: One person is behind the head of the person lying down and holds on tightly to the head, moving it left and right. Do not pull the head.

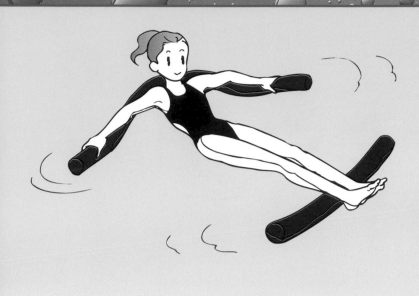

Lie backward on two aqua noodles and relax. One aqua noodle is under your arms and neck, the other under your ankles.

Variation 1

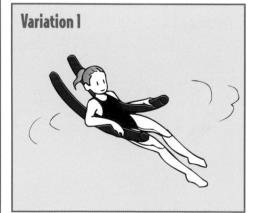

Parallel

Lean on two aqua noodles next to you. Lightly hold onto the aqua noodles.

Variation 2

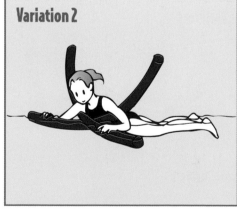

Cross

Lie on two crossed aqua noodles in a prone position. The starting position is very stable because of the high buoyancy of the water.

Stretching

Coordination

Cardio Training

Toning

Fun & Play

Massage & Relaxation

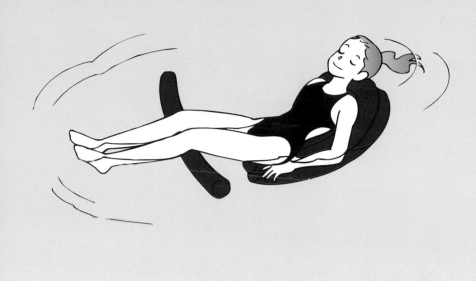

Three aqua noodles: Put two noodles, formed like a ring, under your torso, head and arms. The other one under your knees. You can also use more aqua noodles.

Variation 1

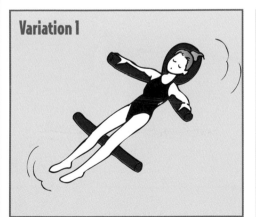

Variation 2

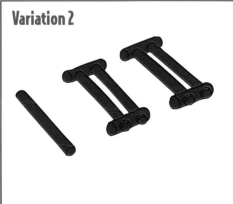

Circle

Relax on three aqua noodles. One is formed like a ring under your head, the second one under your arms and the third one under your knees.

Raft

Put a few aqua noodles with connectors together. This is best suitable for beginners and for therapy because of the good support.

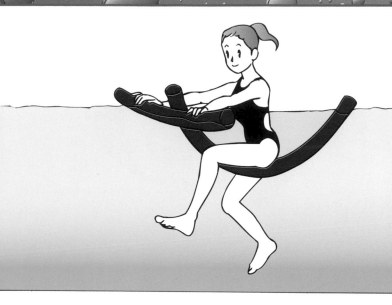

Ride on the aqua noodle. In the picture, the person is riding a bike. Hold on tightly to another aqua noodle with your hands. Now, the starting position is more stable and safer, and you can move easier.

Variation 1

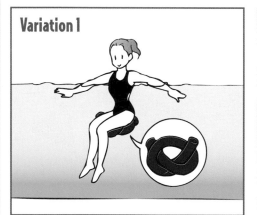

Variation 2

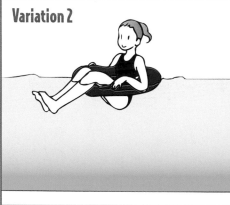

Ball

Sit on the knotted aqua noodle. Using your arms, you go slightly down and up.

Tire

Sit in the aqua noodle formed like ring.

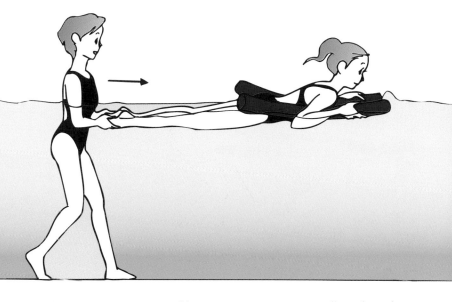

One person is in a prone position and leaning on two aqua noodles. The other person is holding on tightly to the ankles pushing the floating person forward (do not over-extend, hold your stomach in tight). This is a fun and relaxing exercise. You can also massage the feet.

Variation 1

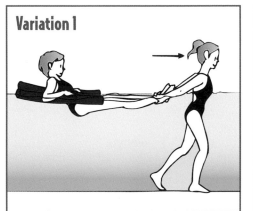

Variation 2

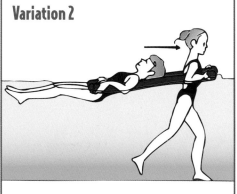

Pull 1

One person is in a supine position. The other person pulls the floating one by the feet. If the person floating lifts up the torso, it works the abdominal muscles. Otherwise, it is good for relaxation.

Pull 2

One person is in a supine position. The partner stands with his back to the person laying down, holds onto the ends of the aqua noodle and pulls him forward. The person lying down can move his legs or just relax.

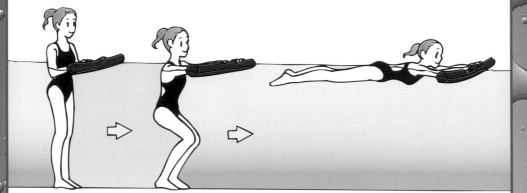

Float on the water in a prone position. Start out in a standing position. Hold on tightly to the aqua noodle with both hands, bend your knees and push yourself into a prone position. It is not important how far you go. Repeat this exercise often. Your face can stay above the water. Do not overextend.

Variation 1

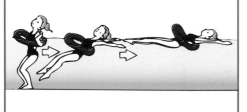

Variation 2

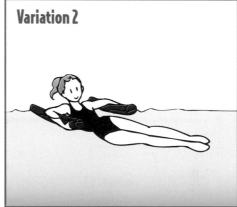

Supine position
The aqua noodle formed like a ring is around your waist. Start out in a standing position. Now, push yourself into a supine position. Extend your arms alongside your head.

Laying on your side
Lie on your side using the two aqua noodles for support. Now, move your legs to stretch your flank.

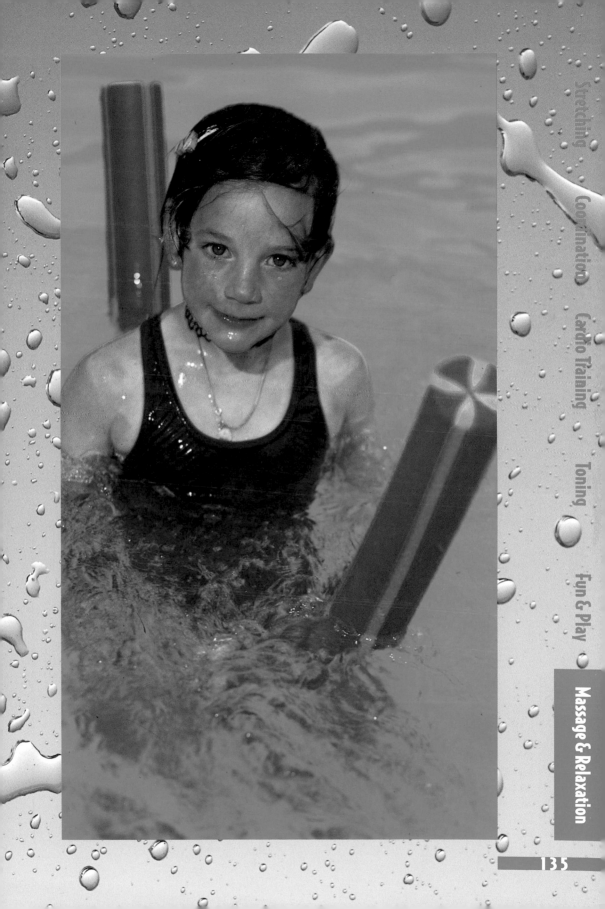

Helpful Tips for the Professional Aqua Instructor

Water Workout with Music

Music plays an important role in every water workout. It motivates participants and the instructor, it helps to structure the lesson and it has a central meaning for the intensity control of the workout.

First, music should be chosen that gives the lesson a theme, for example up to date Charts music, Oldies, Classics, Rock, musicals, Latino music, Techno, Hip Hop or Jazz music. It depends on the taste of the participants and on their and the instructor's goals.

The build-up of the music is as follows:

The basic tempo is named Beats per Minute (BPM). The beat is mostly a four-four time. This means that four beats form a time. There can also be three beats, and then you have a three-four time like the Waltz.

Two times form an eight-phrase. This is also called a measure phrase. Four 8-measure phrases form a major phrase, so 32 BPM.

Consequently, the first beat of the major phrase is also called the big 1. It is emphasized in the music, so one can easily find it. The other three 1s of the 8-measure phrases are also emphasized, but not as much as the big 1. Furthermore the 5 is also emphasized, but again less than the small 1s. The instructor is in need of finding this thread over and over again – even if he has been interrupted.

1 Phrase	Major Phrase			
4 measure Phrases	Measure Phrase	Measure Phrase	Measure Phrase	Measure Phrase
8 Times	Time Time	Time Time	Time Time	Time Time
32 Beats	1-2-3-4-5-6-7-8	1-2-3-4-5-6-7-8	1-2-3-4-5-6-7-8	1-2-3-4-5-6-7-8

Tempo of movement

There are three main tempos for water workouts:

1. Demonstration tempo (4 BPM/movement)
2. Water-specific tempo (2 BPM/movement)
3. Power tempo (1 BPM/movement)

The demonstration tempo is like a slow-motion. It serves the introduction of new movements. The only way to slow down from here is to freeze a position. This pause of the movement helps to improve your technique, your self-perception and the feeling for balance. The water-specific tempo shows the most beneficial effects, because in this tempo the largest functional amplitude of movement is possible. This means strength and flexibility are trained at the same time, so that muscular disharmonism is cleared faster. This is the basic tempo and most of the time applied. The power tempo (also called "land speed") can be a lot of fun, especially for advanced participants. It challenges you more, but the amplitude of the movements is smaller. The range of motion can be reduced to a minimum when you double the speed again, called super-power. After the technique of the movement is clear, this enhancement is pure fun! And finally: Changes of tempo can create a rhythm in your movements.

Choreography

Choreography is a composition and a succession of movements. One can also call it a staging of a course of movements.

First of all one can say that a choreography is also possible in water. It depends on the tempo, the choice and the transformation of the movements. The preconditions are the theoretical basics of music, in order to develop choreography.

A composition of movements can be created for every target group and every fitness level. It merely depends on the build-up, as long as it is slow, exactly explained and often repeated.

The following methods are helpful for practical transformation:

- Add-on-effect: First perform the first step, then the next step. After that the first and the second step are repeated together. Then follows the third step which is repeated together with the first and the second, etc.
- Block-method: Similar to add-on-effect, but is geared to the phases. Initially the first phase is learned, then the second. After that both phases are repeated together until a phrase is full. Then the second phrase is learned and put together with the first, etc.
- Present-effect: The Instructor performs the step sequence alone, and then repeats it together with the group
- 1/2-time-effect: Step sequence is practiced in a half-time
- Insertion-effect: To repeat a familiar step in a different combination
- Pyramid-method: Reduction of the number of repetitions of a movement (16-8-4-2-1)
- Holding pattern: A familiar step is included into a new choreography and at last neglected
- Surprise-effect: Demands spontaneity and creativity, can be planned or not.

In order to create choreography the style of movement, the tempo, the rhythm, the space and the form must be determined. The way a movement is performed shapes the style – for example, whether one chooses soft or hard movements. The tempo, slow or fast, is given by the music. One can vary by using half-tempo, double tempo, by changing tempo and by accentuating. Advanced people can vary the tempo within the group. They can start with new movements simultaneously or after each other.

The dynamics of the movement is of large importance. The movement can be performed softly or very powerfully. The intensity of the movement can be changed punctually or consistently. The modification of strain is also part of the dynamics.

Space can be used in all directions (front, back, side, and diagonal, turned). The center of gravity can be displaced, so every plane and axis can be used. Different ways through your space can be tested. In the water there can be direct, straight and diagonal ways, as well as indirect, curvy, rotational, spiral and zig-zag ways built up in your choreography. For advanced people the line of sight can also be varied by building groups or formations like queues, chains, circles, pyramids, etc.

Also important for your water workout are the foot positions (toe or heels: point and flex). Especially in water, participants tend to leave their heels high not putting them down with every step they do. This is why the basic technique of walking and jogging should be trained very well. In order to achieve healthy and useful effects, the technique-anatomical functional form must be considered when choreography is composed.

The Correct Behavior of a Teacher

- The Aqua Fitness instructors are permanently in the dilemma where to stand in class: In the water or at the edge of the pool? Experts say a combination of both makes sense. Staying in the water has the advantage that the participants are motivated more easily, while the control of the movements and the correct technique is only possible from the edge of the pool.

- The main problem when teaching from the edge of the pool is the difference in the tempo of the movements in water and on land. Water resistance decelerates the movements in the water. The instructor must anticipate the difficulty of the movements and adjust the demonstration of the movements to the possibilities in water. Gravity aggravates the slow demonstration of the movements. Therefore verbal and optical cueing can be helpful.
- Changing positions while teaching also makes sense because beginners often cannot imagine how fast one can move in water and how fast one can see results. When the instructor is in the water for the first ten minutes of a lesson, one can make sure that nobody will get out of the water freezing, because everyone was able to find the right technique and the best level of exercise.

First-aid: Cramp Treatment

A workout in cold water, long workouts or clumsy movements can lead to muscle cramps. They can occur in legs, arms, the torso, and especially in the abs, the fingers or the feet or hands. The part of the body that suffers from cramps the most frequently are the calves and the thighs.

The cramped muscle ought to be stretched. It is advantageous, especially in deep water, to dive the head underneath the water surface, like for the "dead man", and to control breathing while staying calm.

Calf cramp

Pull the toes towards your shin with both hands. Push your knees through.

Thigh Cramp

The knee must be bent. One or two hands pull the toes towards the buttocks.

Abs/Stomach Cramp

Pull both legs towards the torso (like a squat) in a layback position and then stretch fitfully.

Finger Cramp

Pull the fingers together and stretch them apart fitfully.

Cramp Prevention by the Correct Choice of Exercises

Tip: Integrate a flexion of the ankle in your course of movements. It prevents cramps on the backside of your legs and the soles of your feet.

Drinking

Even in the water you must drink enough in order to prevent cramps. That's why we say: "Bring your plastic bottle along with you to the pool and take sips of it throughout your workout."

About the Editor

Michael DeToia

Michael DeToia is a certified physical education teacher, a sports therapist and CEO of DEHAG ACADEMY. The DEHAG ACADEMY, with Michael DeToia as the chairman, has helped to develop many diversified Aquatic Training Programs in Germany and Europe since 1994. Michael's educational programs are characterized by his professionalism, the intensive, cooperative learning atmosphere in group settings and great individual learning outcomes.

Contact: academy@dehag.de

Educational programs and training
DEHAG ACADEMY carries new trends, classical themes of the wellness and group fitness market in the water or on land into effect, developing, supporting and achieving a safe and preventive workout for all fitness levels.

Many national and international cooperations for prevention and rehabilitation between the DEHAG ACADEMY and different universities and educational institutions regarding the topic of health oriented workouts in water have been established.
Contact: academy@dehag.de

Further utilities and products about the aqua noodle
In the meantime plenty useful utilities and products that add to a safe workout in the water have been developed to guarantee fun and efficiency for instructors and sportsmen.

For example, there are 10 waterproof, laminated mini-exercise-programs, derived from this book in a DIN A4 size. They can be used directly at the edge of the pool. For the support of groups there are also 5 different DIN A1 posters concerning different Aqua topics, like "Aqua Muscle Fitness" for Aqua Circuit programs.

Furthermore there is a CD-ROM "Water workout with the noodle" and diverse DVDs for beginners and advanced people. Moreover there is a "starter kit" and also a variety of connectors, as well as the "noodle sticks"- the half noodle. Especially for children there are "play-mats", "action and fun isles" and connectors for the "aqua noodle" and last but not least the "Pool-pony" with funny ears or funny noises when you shake it. The "Aqua-Multi-Gym", a shortened special-noodle with double handles at the ends, has been designed for therapeutic use, beginners and "Aqua-Back-Fit" participants. It provides great help and grip for safe workouts because of its handles.

Service-hotline: ++49 (0)2234-27693 www.dehag.de

Photo & Illustration Credits

Cover Photo: Jump
Cover design: Jens Vogelsang
Photos: BWS, DEHAG
Drawings: DEHAG

Contact the editor: michael.detoia@dehag.de
www.dehag.de